Cognitive Remediation for Brain Injury and Neurological Illness

Marvin H. Podd

Cognitive Remediation for Brain Injury and Neurological Illness

Real Life Changes

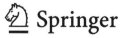 Springer

Marvin H. Podd
National Naval Medical Center
4400 East-West Highway Suite 715
Bethesda, MD 20814
USA
e-mail: marvin.podd@med.navy.mil

ISBN 978-1-4614-1974-7   e-ISBN 978-1-4614-1975-4
DOI 10.1007/978-1-4614-1975-4
Springer New York Dordrecht Heidelberg London

Library of Congress Control Number: 2011940843

© Springer Science+Business Media, LLC 2012
All rights reserved. This work may not be translated or copied in whole or in part without the written permission of the publisher (Springer Science+Business Media, LLC, 233 Spring Street, New York, NY 10013, USA), except for brief excerpts in connection with reviews or scholarly analysis. Use in connection with any form of information storage and retrieval, electronic adaptation, computer software, or by similar or dissimilar methodology now known or hereafter developed is forbidden.
The use in this publication of trade names, trademarks, service marks, and similar terms, even if they are not identified as such, is not to be taken as an expression of opinion as to whether or not they are subject to proprietary rights.

Cover design: eStudio Calamar, Berlin/Figueres

Printed on acid-free paper

Springer is part of Springer Science+Business Media (www.springer.com)

To Don

This book is dedicated to my long-time friend and colleague, Don Seelig, who succumbed to cancer in 2001. We began working together in 1969, entered private practice together in 1976 and began work on NeurXercise about 10 years later. He added his creativity and critical eye to the development of the cognitive remediation exercises and frequently pointed out to me the implications of some of the things I had observed when I did not realize their import for treatment and planning. He co-authored the NeurXercise manual and the first book chapter on using these exercises.

Our relationship was a complex one. He was at once a father and a son, a support and a critic- but always a great help in evaluating myself and my work. Most of my professional and personal growth was a direct product of our interactions, whether they were discussions, arguments or screaming matches. No one could be more exasperating or more endearing. His insights and ability to get to the heart of the matter were unsurpassed. He was fearless and uncompromising when it came to helping others, whether they liked it or not.

He wanted me to write this book for many years and I am glad that I finally have enough material to do so at a level at which he would have approved. I could not have developed the program and my insights without him and the many long discussions we had. I will always miss him, but I hope this book stands as a small testament to him and all that he means to me.

Marvin H. Podd

Preface

The idea of treating the symptoms of brain damage is not new. However, with the advent of Luria's theory (1948, 1966) of brain functioning and his descriptions of its application to remediation of deficits (Luria 1948, 1963) a different approach to treatment became available. With the advent of the microcomputer a more systematic, reliable and objective tool could be used to pursue an approach to teaching compensatory mechanisms. The use of cognitive remediation techniques was initially embraced by neuropsychologists and a number of programs, including those employing microcomputers, flourished. However, difficulties with doing well-controlled studies in the clinical setting along with the publication of a well-controlled study that did not support the efficacy of the treatment led neuropsychologists to become very skeptical. To this day, the majority of brain injury treatment programs in this country focus on the use of prosthetic devices (e.g., keeping a memory log, structuring the day by using a calendar, setting an alarm watch for the time medication is due) rather than helping individuals to use intact brain functions to compensate for deficits. My experience over the past 25 years in the field has been that patients' self-esteem and feeling that they have some control over their lives are more greatly enhanced when they feel that they, themselves, have dealt with their cognitive problems rather than resorting to external mechanisms. In essence, cognitive remediation can provide a normalizing function for both the patient who uses his brain instead of a prosthetic device and for those who interact with the patient and do not observe his compensatory devices. Further, compensatory mechanisms can, at times, serve as basis for a program that restores the "lost" function while prosthetic devices cannot.

The purpose of this book is to help the reader learn more about cognitive remediation and how to develop an effective and efficacious program for patients. After presenting a history of the development of cognitive remediation and the current status of research in the area, the next chapter endeavors to teach treatment planning. Treatment planning is addressed through proper neuropsychological testing and evaluation, with an emphasis on Luria's concepts of alternate functional systems and double dissociation. Brain recovery following the acute stage and the various underlying mechanisms are reviewed. The use of learning theory principles to implement strategies that might potentiate these mechanisms and produce restitution of function is also presented.

The issue of generalization of improved scores to enhanced daily living and better functioning in the occupational and social realms of one's life is next undertaken. The types of assessment that might be used to evaluate these areas and the treatment strategies employed throughout the training are covered. Finally, all of the aspects covered in the book are brought together through the presentation of cases. Cases cover presenting history, evaluation of test results, treatment planning, interventions, progress over the course of treatment, and evaluation of efficacy following cognitive remediation.

As it is my purpose to help others learn how to apply cognitive remediation principles effectively, this last section of the book is a critical and important one. Cases are presented in detail covering numerous cognitive deficits that were remediated, various etiologies of deficit, and different domains of ecological validity that were assessed.

Acknowledgments

I would like to acknowledge the help and support of several people from both the public and private sectors who have made this book possible. Dr. Charles Golden was an early mentor who introduced me to the work of Alexander Luria and the Luria-Nebraska Neuropsychological Battery. This work opened the door to evaluating patients in a way that permitted construction of cognitive remediation programs and informed the basis of my own remediation software, NeurXercise. Dr. Golden was very supportive and encouraging, referring patients for evaluation and follow up treatment. He also encouraged his University colleagues to conduct research with my cognitive remediation software. This eventuated in a doctoral dissertation and a convention poster cited in this volume. Additional help in developing my neuropsychological knowledge came from Drs. Robert Sbordone and Arnold Purisch. Their ideas and insights inspired my thinking about interpreting the meaning of many of the test findings and their implications for treatment.

I owe a debt of gratitude to Dr. Mary Ann Krehbiel, Mrs. Angelique Moran, PO Stephanie Smestad, PO Aaron Treloar and PO Brian Smith who provided me with insights based on their work using the cognitive remediation software. They also provided pre-and/or post-testing on many of the patients treated, some of whom are cited in this book. Dr. Joseph Miller, who ran the EEG lab, facilitated many of our patients getting P300 evoked potentials. Dr. Joseph Boschulte referred from his psychiatric practice many patients who had neurological complications and Dr. William Lightfoot, neurologist, identified many patients who would benefit from cognitive remediation.

Dr. Dennis Reeves introduced me to ANAM, a test I used in evaluating many of the cognitive remediation patients. Also, I would like to thank Dr. Sharat Jain who read over an early draft of the book and provided helpful comments and strong encouragement. Finally, I appreciate Dr. Erik Getka's review of the most recent version of this book and for his helpful editorial suggestions.

Contents

Chapter 1
History of Cognitive Remediation

Scientific understanding of how the brain functions dates back to the late nineteenth century. In 1861, Broca had a patient who lost the ability to express himself and on post mortem was found to have a lesion in the anterior frontal region of the brain. Several more cases were later reported by Broca (1865) with the same finding. The lesioned region was assumed to be the seat of expressive language. Wernicke (1874) found a "receptive language center" in the posterior region of the brain. These findings led to a resurgence of the position promulgated during the previous century by Gall. This has become known as a localizationist or pluripotentialist view of the brain, i.e., the brain was thought to have specialized regions for each behavioral function. Additional support for this position existed with the demonstration that sensory and motor strips contained specific areas that correspond to feeling and movement in particular areas of the body. This localizationist view was challenged by Lashley (1938) and others who believed in mass action or equipotentiality of the brain, i.e., all regions of the brain performed the same functions and that degree of deficit was related to amount of tissue lost rather than location of the damaged tissue.

An equipotentialist, Goldstein (1939), studied brain injured soldiers during World War I and found symptoms of perseveration, inability to anticipate future consequences, figure-ground problems, and loss of abstract reasoning. He believed that loss of the ability to abstract was the hallmark of brain damage. He further believed the cause of this loss was the emotional shock and anxiety connected with loss of brain tissue or reduced function secondary to tissue compromise in the brain. He concluded that treatment should comprise psychotherapy aimed at reducing the emotional reactions to brain damage while permitting the rest of the brain to compensate for disruption of function. The student of functional neuroanatomy may recognize that the symptoms described by Goldstein are classical signs of frontal lobe impairment. This is not a surprise as most of the patients Goldstein saw had sustained frontal head wounds during the war. Thus, Goldstein made some very important early observations about the role of the frontal lobes, but his equipotentialist "blinders" prevented him from seeing the findings for what they actually

M. H. Podd, *Cognitive Remediation for Brain Injury and Neurological Illness*,
DOI: 10.1007/978-1-4614-1975-4_1, © Springer Science+Business Media, LLC 2012

were. It remained for Alexander Luria to clarify the nature of brain functioning and identify the roles and functions of various brain regions and the critical role played by interactive functional systems or what are now referred to as neural networks.

During World War II Luria saw most of the brain-injured soldiers in Russia as they were sent to the Burdenko Institute of Neurosurgery in Moscow where he was affiliated. He had worked with Pavlov and Vygotsky and was highly respected in Russian scientific circles. He developed a theory of brain functioning (Luria 1948, 1966, 1973) that bridged the gap between equipotentialism and pluripotentialism. He acknowledged that there were regions of the brain that were involved in specific functions, but that it was also true that the brain was capable of spontaneously reorganizing such that a different area could take over the function of a damaged region. A major contribution was that behavior was the product of functional systems or the interaction of diverse brain areas. Damage to any area involved in a specific functional system could reduce effective functioning in the target behavior without disrupting the function altogether (consistent with the observations of the equipotentialists). Further, one could detect the region of dysfunction (consistent with the pluriopotentialists) by assessing the way the target behavior was disrupted. For example, when short-term memory is disrupted, is the impairment for auditory, visual, tactile, and/or kinesthetic material? This would be critical as the temporal lobe processes auditory material, the occipital lobe processes visual stimuli, the parietal lobe processes tactile material, and the posterior parietal region processes kinesthetic material. In addition, use of alternate functional systems could be taught when the cause of the damage was analyzed. Thus, if the memory problem was auditory, while visual and kinesthetic systems were intact, the patient could be taught to learn and remember using the intact modalities rather than the premorbidly preferred modality. Similarly, arithmetic problems could be analyzed to determine if they were due to not understanding the meaning of numbers, loss of calculation ability, or problems with the spatial aspect of arithmetic. In his evaluations Luria used a system of double dissociation. This involved presentation of the same tasks with single differences, usually in the input or output modality. Thus, one might read a question before answering it, hear the question without reading it, answer the question verbally, or point to the correct answer. Through a series of such questions and tasks Luria was able to determine which modalities or skills were impaired and therefore which parts of the brain were compromised. Once Luria's system of double dissociation was employed to determine the regions of the brain and the specific behaviors that were disrupted and intact, a treatment plan could be devised to develop and teach alternate functional systems (Luria 1948, 1963).

Although Luria published his theory and findings during and shortly after World War II, they were not translated into English for another 15–20 years. American neuropsychologists dismissed Luria's work because it could not be tested empirically, as his tests by definition were individualized rather than standardized and therefore were not subject to the group research designs these psychologists demanded for tests of scientific validity. When a standardized battery was developed to allow for this type of research, this group criticized the test as not representing Luria's approach because the Russian neuropsychologist had insisted evaluation had to be individualized and not standardized.

Nonetheless, the Luria-Nebraska Neuropsychological Battery (LNNB; Golden et al. 1979, 1995, 1999) validated many of Luria's claims for his theory and approach to neuropsychological assessment (Golden, Warren and Espe-Pfeiffer, 1999). Most of the criticisms of the testing battery were based on an insufficient understanding of Luria's theory. The test was criticized on statistical grounds but subsequent analyses found it to be reliable and valid for a variety of clinical populations (Moses and Maruish 1990). Many of the criticisms of the test were nonempirical criticisms. Moses and Maruish report later empirical tests of those criticisms and that research did not support the detractors of the LNNB. The major exception was that the alternate form of the test (LNNB II) was not a true alternate form and should not be used as such (Moses and Maruish 1991). Although the potential for developing cognitive remediation programs from the results of the Battery was clear, research was focused almost exclusively on the assessment aspects of the instrument.

Interest in treating cognitive deficits following brain injury was, however, beginning to grow around the time that the Luria-Nebraska was developed. Craine and Gudeman (1981) published their book on neurotraining, in which they describe their approach to cognitive remediation and recommend "off-the-shelf" games that could be adapted for helping brain damaged patients improve their cognitive functioning. With the advent of the personal computer, Lynch (1979) recommended Atari games, and later Apple II games, that could be helpful to cognitively impaired patients.

Neuropsychologists began to develop their own computer-assisted cognitive remediation programs and make them available to other professionals (e.g., Ben-Yishay et al. 1987; Bracy 1985; Gianutsos and Klitzner 1981). Although great interest blossomed at this time, research was not conducted to a great degree and neuropsychologists became skeptical of the efficacy of cognitive remediation. One of the more significant blows dealt to cognitive remediation at that time was a well-controlled study by Ponsford and Kinsella (1988), which demonstrated that apparent improvement in acute head injured patients in a rehabilitation program was a product of spontaneous recovery rather than treatment. Amazingly, no one seemed to recall that Von Monakow had reported in the early 1900s that spontaneous recovery takes place in the acute phase. Cognitive remediation could only be meaningfully tested in patients who had residual deficits following the acute phase. Research began to slowly accumulate and in 1999 an NIH conference concluded that there was support and promise for cognitive remediation as an effective treatment tool although more Class I studies (i.e., prospective, double-blind, randomized designs) were desirable. Cicerone et al. (2000, 2005) reviewed the cognitive remediation literature for head injury and stroke patients and looked at whether the patients in the studies were in the acute or post-acute phase of recovery. They found significant support from Class I as well as Class II and III studies. The preponderance of the evidence supported the efficacy of cognitive remediation for attentional deficits, visual perceptual difficulties, memory problems, and executive dysfunction. There was suggestive support for the generalization of improvement on tests to ecologically valid measures. Almost 80% of the Class I studies demonstrated superiority of cognitive remediation compared to other treatments while the remainder showed equal amounts of improvement to other treatments. Clearer evidence of generalization and ecological validity was demonstrated by Cicerone (2002), and Podd and Krehbiel (2006). Concrete daily living skill improvements following cognitive remediation with post-acute patients were found when such improvements were not seen in control groups. Klonoff et al. (2010) demonstrated that 50.5% of their patients receiving cognitive remediation focusing on process variables and metacognitive skills were able to be cleared for driving a vehicle. Klonoff's group (2007) also demonstrated that this approach led to over 80% of their patients returning to paid employment or school. Germano and Capellini (2008) demonstrated that dyslexic students who performed poorly on auditory processing and phonological awareness compared to good readers were able to score similarly to the controls (good readers) following treatment with an audio-visual remediation program.

Chapter 2
The Role of Assessment in Treatment Planning

Neuropsychological assessment is critical to the planning of cognitive remediation and forms the basis of the plan and interventions to be carried out. Discussion of the major cognitive domains and the tests used to assess them constitutes the bulk of this chapter.

Before describing the cognitive domains and the tests that sample them, there are a few important concepts worth repeating and expanding upon. The concept of functional systems is a particularly useful one for cognitive remediation (Luria 1963, 1973, 1980). Luria posits that behavior is the product of the interaction of different brain regions. Each region contributes different behavioral links to the chain that comprises the target behavior. If any link in the chain of regions is damaged, the behavior will be disrupted. However, the nature of the disruption will be distinct, depending on the link that is dysfunctional. For example, responding to a telephone ringing could be disrupted because it is not heard, the phone could not be found (i.e., located in space), kinesthetic guidance of hand to phone was disrupted, etc. Thus, identification of the functional system used to accomplish a particular behavior and the link(s) in that chain that are dysfunctional comprises the initial step in evaluation for treatment planning.

Once the functional system and its components have been identified, alternate functional systems can be constructed that will allow the patient to perform the behavior while bypassing the dysfunctional link(s). This provides one or more compensatory systems that can be learned and practiced. For example, if memory complaints are due to auditory memory disruption in the presence of intact visual memory, the patient can be taught several different compensatory strategies. He/she may create visual images or pictures of the information to be recalled, read the information rather than listening to lectures, or take notes to be read later.

In performing any evaluation and especially one for cognitive remediation planning, the assessor should utilize "double dissociation." This concept refers to a method of evaluation in which the same test item or task is presented in slightly different forms in order to determine the specific cognitive skills that are intact and those that are impaired. In Luria's terms, links in the functional system are

M. H. Podd, *Cognitive Remediation for Brain Injury and Neurological Illness*,
DOI: 10.1007/978-1-4614-1975-4_2, © Springer Science+Business Media, LLC 2012

replaced by others in order to determine those that are functional and those that are not. An alternate functional system is then identified that permits the task to be accomplished by using an intact system rather than the previously used one that is now dysfunctional. For example, the same question might be asked (auditory input), then be presented in writing (visual input) and the answer might be given verbally (expressive language output) and by pointing (motor output). If the question can be answered in one input modality but not the other, the patient may have a deficit in the modality in which he/she performed inadequately. If the patient cannot answer the question regardless of modality, the problem may lie in the cognitive domain of the question (e.g., reasoning, memory). Similarly, if the patient responds correctly in one output channel but not the other, the evaluator must consider the possibility that there is a deficit in that channel. If neither channel yields a correct response, the possibility must be considered that the cognitive domain is impaired. In each instance the incorrect response suggests a hypothesis to be tested with additional items that will eventually lead to the conclusion of the actual deficits requiring remediation. This is the approach described by Luria (1963, 1973, 1980) and incorporated into the Luria-Nebraska Neuropsychological Battery (Golden et al. 1979, 1995).

The rest of the chapter will be devoted to outlining the cognitive domains usually assessed by neuropsychologists and the tests most often used to assess those domains. Further, sub groupings under each larger domain will be identified and the tests sensitive to them will be described and discussed.

Cognitive Domains

There are a number of major cognitive domains that should be assessed in determining what skills need remediation. Attention and concentration are important domains that need careful evaluation. Tests should be given that assess focused, sustained, alternating, selective, and divided attention. Processing speed should also be assessed. Rhythm and pitch perception are likewise usually examined. Another domain is sensorimotor functioning. This includes fine and gross motor ability and speed, graphesthesia (identification of information traced on the skin), and stereognosis (identification of objects by touch). The domain of visual perception includes visual naming and spatial ability. Constructional praxis is an area related to visual perception and sensorimotor functioning and involves organizing "elements in correct spatial relationships so that they form an entity" (Benton and Tranel 1993). This includes ability to draw or in some other way construct an object or design. Language should also be assessed in a neuropsychological battery. This includes expressive and receptive speech. Memory should be evaluated for verbal and nonverbal material on an immediate and delayed basis. Auditory, visual, and motor input and output channels should be assessed. Simple and complex information and long and short delays should be explored when evaluating memory. Intellectual functioning should be tested for verbal and nonverbal materials.

Premorbid IQ and academic performance are very helpful in determining the degree to which the current functioning is below expectation. Auditory, visual, and motor input and output channels should be assessed on intelligence measures. Executive functions include problem solving, convergent/divergent thinking, ability to shift set, multitasking, generation and testing of hypotheses, ability to perform novel tasks, impulse control, and use of good judgment.

Some tests that tap into the cognitive domains and their various subdivisions follow. These will be described in terms of input–output characteristics to help the evaluator to think about which tests to use for a specific assessment. Using a variety of modalities for input and output allows for double dissociation and better, more specific, treatment planning. Appendices A-I summarize the salient characteristics of each test to help in making the double dissociations necessary for treatment planning.

Attention and Concentration

Focused Attention

Ability to briefly focus one's attention is assessed with a variety of tasks. Auditory focused attention can be assessed with Digit Span Forward from the Wechsler Adult Intelligence Scale-Third or Fourth Edition (WAIS III, WAIS IV) or the Wechsler Memory Scale-Third Edition (WMS III), the 0-second delay condition on Auditory Consonant Trigrams, the Rhythm Scale and Word Repetition Factor Scale of the Luria-Nebraska Neuropsychological Battery (LNNB), the Seashore Rhythm Scale and Speech Sounds Perception Test from the Halstead-Reitan Neuropsychological Battery (HRNB), and the Token Test. Auditory input is numerical on Digits Forward, tonal on LNNB Rhythm and Seashore Rhythm, and verbal on Auditory Consonant Trigrams, the Token Test, Word Repetition Factor Scale, and Speech Sounds. Output is verbal on Digit Span, Trigrams, most of LNNB Rhythm, Seashore Rhythm, and Word Repetition. Output is motoric for Speech Sounds (i.e., underlining the correct answer in a multiple choice format.), Token Test (carrying out the verbal command) and a few LNNB Rhythm items (i.e., tapping of rhythms).

Visual focused attention can be assessed with Spatial Span Forward from the WMS III, the sample trial of the Trail Making Test (Part A), and the Word and Color trials of the Stroop Color and Word Test. Spatial Span is a visual-nonverbal analog to Digit Span. Input is visual and output is motoric. The sample trial of Trails A is brief enough to be a good measure of focused attention. Input is visual and output is motoric. The Stroop trials usually take about a minute and as such, have focused and sustained attention elements. Reading each word requires focused attention and continuously performing the task for approximately a minute requires sustained attention for that period of time. The color trial is visual-nonverbal input with a verbal output. The word trial is visual–verbal input with verbal output.

Sustained Attention

Keeping one's attention focused for a longer time is tapped by the Conner's Continuous Performance Test, the Running Memory subtest of the 1990s version of Automated Neuropsychological Assessment Metric (ANAM) and the current version of ARES, Visual Search and Attention Test (VSAT), the Paced Auditory Serial Addition Test (PASAT), and the Color and Word trials of the Stroop. Input is visual for all but the PASAT, which is auditory. Output is motoric on all but the PASAT, which is verbal. Visual input is verbal on the Conner's, ANAM, ARES, and Stroop Word. Visual input is colors on Stroop Color and VSAT. Auditory input is numeric on PASAT.

Visual sustained attention is assessed for about 15 min on the Conner's and about 5 min on ANAM and ARES. These are computer administered and scores are saved in patient files. The Stroop and VSAT assess visual sustained attention for about a minute. Auditory sustained attention is assessed on PASAT. Fifty (Levin modification of the PASAT) or sixty numbers (Gronwall's original test) are presented at a rate of 2.4 seconds between stimuli on the first trial, 2.0 seconds on the second trial, 1.6 seconds on the third trial, and 1.2 seconds on the fourth trial. Thus, auditory sustained attention is evaluated over approximately a minute or two. Processing speed plays a major role on this test.

Alternating Attention

The ability to shift attention between tasks is assessed on the Trail Making Test (Part B), ANAM and ARES Running Memory, Conner's CPT, LNNB items (e.g., alternating tapping patterns with right and left hand, alternating motor movements of right and left hand, copying alternating figure), and letter cancelation tasks with target shifting every other line. Input is visual for Trails B, ANAM, ARES, the Conner's CPT, letter cancelation and LNNB items. Input is auditory on an LNNB item requiring tapping of rhythm played on a tape recorder. Output is motoric on all of the above tests. Stimuli are verbal on ANAM, ARES, the Conner's and most cancelation tasks. They are verbal and numeric on Trails B. Stimuli are nonverbal on the LNNB items. Specifically, they are hand movements, tapping patterns, and copying drawings.

Divided Attention

Multitasking is evaluated on Auditory Consonant Trigrams, Digit Span Backwards, and Spatial Span Backwards. Input is auditory for Trigrams and Digits Backward and visual for Spatial Span Backwards. Output is verbal for Trigrams and Digits but motoric for Spatial Span.

Trigrams requires the patient to remember three-letter combinations while counting backwards by threes from designated numbers. The amount of time that the individual has to multitask is varied over three time periods. Each three-letter combination is accompanied by a designated number from which the subject must count backwards by threes and by a delay period that must elapse before having to repeat the trigram (9, 18, or 36 seconds).

Digits Backwards involves holding the digits in mind while trying to repeat them in reverse order. Spatial Span Backwards requires the subject to remember the sequence that the evaluator pointed to while trying to point to the stimuli in reverse order. Both Spans require maintenance of the forward sequence in order to perform the string in reverse order.

Selective Attention

This involves screening out irrelevant stimuli and attending to the designated target. Letter cancelation tasks require selective attention, especially when they include complexities such as canceling the target letter only when preceded or followed by a specific letter. Unintentionally, the Speech Sounds Perception Test is so poorly recorded that it provides a selective attention element. The same is true of the old LNNB Rhythm tape, which has been subsequently re-recorded.

Letter cancelation involves visual input and motor output. Speech Sounds and LNNB Rhythm involve auditory input. Output is motor for Speech Sounds and verbal/motor for LNNB Rhythm.

Processing Speed

Speed of performance and reaction time are measures of processing speed. Tests that measure this include Stroop, PASAT, the Conner's, ANAM and ARES Running Memory, LNNB Speed scale, letter cancelation tests, and Trails A. Input is visual for all but PASAT (auditory) and LNNB. The LNNB includes processing speed in the motor, tactile, visual, verbal-expressive, and mathematical calculation domains. The raw score is converted into a T score so as to be comparable to all other scales on the LNNB. It is especially useful to compare this score to the "power" score, which is accuracy on the same items as are assessed for speed.

Perception

Visual Scanning and Tracking

Closely related to visual focused attention is visual scanning. It is an element in both parts of the Trail Making Test. The Visual Search and Attention Test (VSAT) as well as other cancelation tasks also tap into this area. Picture Arrangement

(WAIS III) and Picture Completion from WAIS III and IV require careful scanning for important details. Items on the LNNB have visual scanning components (e.g., description of pictures, quickly reading a paragraph, identifying specific themes depicted, attending to visual details to help in correct visual sequencing.) Digit Symbol on WAIS III and Coding on WAIS IV, like all hand–eye coordination tests, have a scanning component.

Input is obviously always visual. As previously mentioned, output is motoric on Trails and VSAT. It is also motoric on Digit Symbol, Coding, and the Picture Arrangement items of the Luria and WAIS III and/or IV. Output for other visual scanning items on the LNNB and Picture Completion is verbal.

Spatial Organization

Orientation in space is assessed on the Tactile Performance Test (TPT). This test is given while the subject is blindfolded and he/she must place the shapes in the proper slots with the proper orientations through the tactile and motor modes. Grooved Pegboard requires the proper spatial orientation of the pegs in order for them to be placed onto the board. Clock drawings require proper spatial placement of the hands of the clock to designate the time requested. The Hooper Visual Organization Test presents pictures that have been cut into pieces and placed in different spatial orientations. The subject is to identify the depicted object by reorienting the pieces mentally. The LNNB has items that necessitate imposing three dimensions on two-dimensional pictures, and mentally rotating squares to match a target. The Raven's Progressive Matrices requires identification of the correct piece of an abstract puzzle-like design containing spatially variant lines. Porteus Mazes require finding one's way through mazes presented on paper. WAIS III and IV Block Design and WAIS III Object Assembly also require intact spatial organization for rapid, correct performance.

The TPT involves tactile input and motor output. There is an incidental memory portion of the test that requires the patient to make a drawing of the board with the correct spatial placement of the various figures. Grooved Pegboard has a visual input and motor/spatial output. The Hooper has visual input and verbal output. Clock drawings have a verbal input (the instruction) and a motor/spatial output. The LNNB items have a visual input and verbal output. Matrices, Mazes, Block Design, and Object Assembly have a visual input and motoric output (pointing to the correct piece, tracing with a pencil the path through the maze, constructing the depicted design, putting the pieces of the puzzle together).

Rhythm and Pitch Perception

This involves the ability to perceive and produce differences in auditory pitch and rhythmic patterns. The Seashore Rhythm Test from the HRNB and the Rhythm Scale from the LNNB are the best known and most widely used measures of this aspect of perception. The Seashore requires comparisons of tonal patterns and the subject must determine whether the two patterns played on a tape recorder are the same or different. There are similar items on the LNNB but it also includes a wider range of items to assess the target skills. These include tapping rhythms, identifying which tones are higher in pitch, reproducing relative differences in pitches, and singing melodies.

Input is auditory for both Rhythm scales. For the Seashore the input is always tonal patterns. For the LNNB it may be tonal, tapped rhythms, or verbal instructions. Output is verbal for the Seashore. Output varies for the LNNB. Some items include verbal/vocal output. The verbal/vocal output may be tonal productions or words. Other output may be motoric (e.g., tapping rhythms) or verbal (e.g., reporting the higher pitch).

Sensorimotor Skill

Fine and Gross Motor Skill and Speed

The LNNB Motor scale includes factors for fine motor speed and drawing speed, oral praxis, kinesthesis-based movement, and spatial-based movement, as well as gross motor items. Tasks involve hand and finger movements, arm movement, oral motor performance, manual motor speed, and copying/drawing. Drawings will be discussed under the constructional praxis section. Perdue Pegboard and Grooved Pegboard are fine motor skill and speed tests. There is a gross motor aspect to the Tactile Performance Test (TPT) from the HRNB. Finger oscillation is a fine motor speed test and strength of grip is a gross motor strength task, both from the HRNB.

Output is motoric on all tests. Input on the LNNB Motor scale is usually auditory-verbal or visual-nonverbal. The pegboard tests, finger oscillation, and grip strength have auditory-verbal input (instructions). The TPT utilizes tactile input.

Sensory Perception

The HRNB Sensory Perception Examination evaluates finger, hand and face sensation, hearing and auditory perception, and visual fields. Bilateral stimulation helps identify suppressions, which are indicative of lateralized brain damage. The LNNB Tactile scale includes sensory perception of the hands to sharp/dull and hard/soft stimulation, finger sensation discrimination, graphesthesia, and stereognosis.

On the Sensory Perception Exam input is usually tactile but there are items that have auditory or visual input. Output is usually verbal. The LNNB Tactile scale involves tactile input. Output is verbal or motor. The LNNB Motor scale includes some tactile input items.

Stereognosis

This involves tactile identification of stimuli. The TPT requires the blindfolded subject to place large wooden shapes into openings of the same shape on a board. The Sensory Perception Examination has small plastic shapes for tactile identification. The Tactile scale on the LNNB uses common objects encountered in daily life that are to be identified by the blindfolded subject.

Input is always tactile. Output is motoric on TPT and verbal on Sensory Perception and LNNB.

Constructional Praxis

This relates to visuoconstructional skill. Specifically, it involves the "capacity to organize elements in correct spatial relationships so that they form an entity" (Benton and Tranel 1993). It includes drawing, and constructing, producing, or reproducing designs. The Reitan-Indiana Aphasia Screening Test, from the HRNB, includes items on which the subject draws a Greek Cross and a key. The LNNB includes drawing a mildly complex figure and geometric shapes. Visual Reproduction from WMS III and IV provides moderately complex designs and the Rey Complex figure is a highly complex design. Block Design from WAIS III and IV requires the subject to use blocks to construct depicted designs. Clock drawings are also measures of constructional praxis. On LNNB clock drawings the subject has to draw the hands of the clock on blank clock faces to depict designated times.

Output is always motoric on tests of constructional praxis. On Aphasia Screening input is audioverbal. On the LNNB input is audioverbal or visual. On Block Design input is visual. For clock drawings input is verbal. These tests therefore make for a very convenient way to use double dissociation to determine whether construction problems are differentially affected by audioverbal or visual input.

Language

Expressive Speech

Motor speech or ability to express oneself is tapped by the LNNB Expressive Speech Scale and the HRNB Aphasia Screening Test. The Boston Naming Test and Controlled Oral Word Association Test (COWAT) are other widely used measures. The Thurstone Word Fluency Test is useful for examining double dissociation when given in conjunction with the COWAT.

The LNNB scale includes word and sound repetition and reading aloud. Aphasia Screening includes verbal repetition and generation of a verbal explanation of a sentence. On Boston Naming the patient is shown drawings and must respond with the name of the depicted object. Phonemic and categorical cues may be provided if the individual fails to correctly name the object in the drawing. The task on the COWAT is to verbally generate as many words beginning with a prescribed letter over a designated period of time. The Thurstone is a similar task except that the individual writes the words rather than saying them.

Output is verbal on all but the Thurstone, which is motoric. Input on LNNB and Aphasia Screening is audioverbal or visual. Input on Boston Naming is visual while it is audioverbal for COWAT and the Thurstone.

Receptive Speech

This relates to verbal comprehension in the auditory modality when no sensory deficits are present. That is, the subject has no hearing problems but may have difficulty understanding the spoken language. The Receptive Speech Scale on the LNNB and both Speech Sounds Perception Test and Aphasia Screening on HRNB are measures of this area. The Token Test also assesses receptive speech. The LNNB evaluates phonemic discrimination, understanding of concepts, and relationships, and ability to follow simple commands. Aphasia Screening includes understanding and following directions. Speech Sounds involves phonemic discrimination. The Token Test requires the subject to follow a set of instructions.

Input is always audioverbal. On the LNNB input may add a visual stimulus to the audioverbal instruction. Output is verbal or motoric. Aphasia Screening output may be verbal or motoric. Output on Speech Sounds and the Token Test is motoric.

Memory

Memory may be subdivided in a number of different ways. One may consider the input channel. For example, there is the verbal–nonverbal dimension and sensory input channel (e.g., auditory, visual, tactile). One may consider immediate and delayed memory. Delayed memory may be subdivided into short-term or long-term and may involve seconds, minutes, hours, or years of delay. The characteristics of the material to be retrieved may be considered. There is contextual (e.g., a story or meaningful association) versus noncontextual material (e.g., a list of unrelated words or nonsense sounds). Declarative and procedural memory refer to conscious and unconscious processes, respectively (conscious recall of learned material like who wrote a certain book versus overlearned, automatic behaviors like driving). Semantic memory may be contrasted with episodic memory even though both are declarative. Episodic memory refers to retrieving information about one's life while semantic memory refers to knowledge about the world outside of oneself. Depending on the question and patient any of these distinctions may be useful, even though they often overlap with each other. Finally, method of access (e.g., free recall, cued recall, recognition) is salient in determining the stage at which memory might be impaired, i.e., encoding, consolidation/storage, or retrieval.

Verbal Memory

Logical Memory I from the Wechsler Memory Scale (WMS III and IV) comprises stories read aloud to the examinee by the tester. It is contextual, declarative, semantic, and involves immediate memory. Logical Memory II is the retrieval of information included in that story after 30 minutes (i.e., delayed memory). The LNNB contains a story for immediate and delayed recall (15 minutes).

List learning can be assessed on the California Verbal Learning Test (CVLT-II), Rey Auditory Verbal Learning Test (AVLT), Cued Selective Reminding Test, the LNNB and the WMS III/IV. Each has an immediate memory component, a learning component (except for WMS IV), and a delay (30 min for all but the LNNB which has a 15-min delay). Only the CVLT-II provides context (words can be categorized) whereas the others are noncontextual. There are 16 words on the CVLT-II and Selective Reminding, 15 words on the AVLT, 12 words on the WMS III/IV Word List, and 7 words on the LNNB. All are declarative and semantic.

Verbal Paired Associates is a WMS III/IV subtest in which the examinee learns word pairings. Memory under interference conditions is assessed by Auditory Consonant Trigrams and LNNB. A distraction is interpolated between stimulus and response on these tests. Trigrams require the examinee to count backwards by 3's while attempting to retain the three letters he/she was asked to remember. On the LNNB two sets of stimuli are read and the subject is asked to repeat the first one and then the second one. This procedure allows for evaluation of retroactive and proactive interference effects. AVLT and CVLT interference trials also examine proactive and retroactive interference. Interference trials involve the presentation of a second list after the first list has been practiced several times. Following this, the examinee is asked to recall the items on this second list. Immediately thereafter, he/she is asked to recall the words from the first list.

Delayed memory is assessed on the LNNB for 15 minutes to 3 hours of delay. Trigram delays are 9, 18, and 36 seconds. The other tests have a 30-minutes delay.

Input is audioverbal in all instances. It also includes visual and spatial input on Selective Reminding. Output is vocal on all of the above verbal memory tests.

Nonverbal Memory

These tests include tactile, visual, and spatial learning and retrieval. The TPT has two memory measures. Following learning with each hand separately and both hands together, the examinee is asked to draw the form board and the shapes that were on it. The client is scored for the number of forms recalled and correct spatial placement. There is an LNNB item that asks for recall of shapes that had been felt during the stereognosis item.

Visual memory is tapped by the Rey Complex Figure, Visual Reproduction I and II from the WMS III/IV, and the Luria Complex Figure. The Luria figure is the least complex, WMS figures are moderately complex, and Rey is highly complex. Patients may do well on the simple and moderately complex figures and poorly on the highly complex one. This is an important double dissociation to make. The degree of visual memory deficits, when it is likely to be a problem, and the underlying nature of the deficits may all be examined by using the three figures. To minimize interference effects, the tests should be given as far apart from each other as possible, even on separate days if that is feasible.

The LNNB contains visual memory items for immediate and delayed response. Figural Memory and Visual Paired Associates are WMS-R subtests. The former is a recognition test and the latter is a figure–color learning paradigm.

The tactile modality serves as input for TPT and the LNNB stereognosis recall item. Output is motoric for TPT recall and verbal for LNNB. The complex figures involve visual input and motoric output. LNNB visual memory items have motoric and verbal output channels. Output for Figural Memory is motoric and for Visual Paired Associates it is verbal.

Method of Accessing Data

If one plans to remediate memory, it is imperative to determine whether the memory problem lies in the encoding, storage, or retrieval stage of memory. By varying the method by which the information is retrieved, the examiner may gather some useful information about this important question. Some people may need to learn by using multiple channels or encoding does not take place. Others may need to use one channel or avoid one or more channels if encoding is to take place. Immediate performance reflects encoding. Learning from repeated exposures relates to consolidation or storage. If information is encoded and stored, it can be retrieved via one or more methods.

Free recall is assessed on the above list learning tasks after the learning trials and after a delay. It is also assessed on the complex figure drawings immediately and after a delay. Recall of the forms and their placement on TPT and of the objects on the LNNB stereognostic test also qualify for evaluating free recall. Logical Memory assesses free recall after a 30-min delay while the LNNB story has a 15-min delay.

Very often information is stored but the patient cannot retrieve it through free recall. In these instances stimulus cuing or recognition demonstrates that the information was in fact retained. This is especially useful in examining for Alzheimer's Dementia in which most information does not get encoded and stored. Patients who remember information poorly through free recall but recognize it at a much better level are unlikely to be suffering from Alzheimer's disease. Cued recall is assessed on Verbal Paired Associates from WMS III/IV, Visual Paired

Associates from WMS-R, and Selective Reminding. Cued recall is optional on Logical Memory II of WMS III/IV.

There are recognition trials on the Rey Complex Figure, Visual Reproduction, AVLT, LNNB delayed memory section, Logical Memory, Word Lists, and Verbal Paired Associates. Both cues and recognition are included in the Cued Selective Reminding Test.

Intellectual Functioning

WAIS III/IV assesses a range of intellectual skills, producing indices of Verbal Comprehension, Perceptual Organization, Working Memory, and Processing Speed. Estimated IQ range within a 95% Confidence Interval is also reported. This is the most commonly used IQ test. Shorter tests of estimated IQ include the Wechsler Abbreviated Scale of Intelligence (WASI), Shipley Institute of Living Scale (SILS), and the Kaufman Brief Intelligence Test (KBIT). The LNNB Intellectual Processes scale yields an estimated IQ as well. Premorbid IQ may be estimated from the North American Adult Reading Test (NAART). This test employs nonphonetic words that are usually mispronounced unless they are in the subject's premorbid vocabulary. A premorbid IQ estimate can be made from the words that are part of the premorbid vocabulary. The Barona Index uses demographics to estimate premorbid IQ and the Armed Forces Qualification Test (AFQT), taken by all armed forces enlistees, can be converted into an estimated IQ. Following a head injury, the AFQT estimate can be compared with the obtained IQ score.

Tests are usually divided into verbal and nonverbal ones. They may include overlearned skills, such as vocabulary, and nonverbal problem solving skills, such as continuing a progression or matrix reasoning. Most IQ tests do not sample executive functions to a great extent so this will be covered in a separate section.

Of import for the neuropsychologist and treatment planner is that IQ tests are notoriously unreliable as indicators of lateralized brain damage. While a simplistic approach would suggest that poor performance on verbal relative to nonverbal subtests reflects left hemisphere injury and vice versa, this is not the case in practice. The tests are complex and require careful double dissociation to determine why they were performed inadequately. Premorbid education and functioning is often critical in diagnosing why an individual scored a particular way. A head injury patient who scores poorly on Arithmetic and Digit Span will have a Verbal IQ and Working Memory deficit score on the test, but this could be due to premorbid Math Learning Disability or Math Phobia and be unrelated to the head injury or verbal, attentional, or left hemisphere functioning.

It is assumed that the reader is most acquainted with IQ tests more so than any of the other tests herein discussed. Therefore, I will proceed to Academic functioning.

Academic Functioning

Academic functioning is correlated with intelligence, but some individuals may have academic deficits unrelated to brain injury. This may be due to learning disability, poor school attendance, math or reading phobia, etc. It is therefore important to determine whether basic academic skills are in line with intellectual functioning. The LNNB assesses basic capabilities in reading, writing, spelling, and arithmetic. The WRAT-3 and 4 assesses basic arithmetic, spelling, and reading. A more thorough evaluation can be accomplished with the Woodcock-Johnson III (WJ III) or the WIAT II and III. WJ III and WIAT II/III cover reading, math, oral language, and written language.

The LNNB has auditory and visual-spatial input in each area while output is verbal for reading, motoric for writing, and both verbal and motoric for spelling and arithmetic. WRAT-3/4 math is visual input and motor output; spelling and reading have visual input and verbal output. WJ III reading has visual-verbal input with verbal and motoric output; math input is visual and output motoric; oral language has visual-pictorial input and verbal output; written language includes auditory and visual input with motoric output. On WIAT II/III reading input is visual and output is verbal and motoric; math input is verbal and visual and output is verbal and motoric; written language includes audioverbal input and motoric output; oral language has audioverbal and visual-verbal input with verbal output.

Executive Functions

Executive functions, according to Luria (1966, 1980), involve the programming, regulating, and verifying of mental activity. Lezak (1995) wrote that executive functions include volition, planning, purposive action, and effective performance. Tests that sample this domain cover ability to shift set, ability to perform novel tasks, problem solving, impulse control, and judgment.

Set Shifting

Once the subject has determined a correct course of action, the action is followed until feedback suggests that a new course is required. In Luria's terms, there has been programming until the program is no longer verified as correct. At that time the individual must shift set and try a new response and generate new hypotheses until a new correct solution is verified. This is one type of set shifting task and it will be the first discussed.

The Category Test from the HRNB presents a target and four choices from which the subject must choose the correct answer. The patient keeps generating answers consistent with the principle determined to produce correct feedback.

At some point the principle changes and the subject has to shift set in order to determine what the new principle will be that will generate positive feedback. The testee is provided with constant reminders that the principle may change. In contrast, the Wisconsin Card Sort does not cue the examinee that the principle may change. Thus, this test places a greater emphasis on ability to shift set with minimal feedback and direction, other than the information regarding correctness of the response. Input is visual and output motoric on both tests.

Another type of task that requires shifting of set is one in which the individual must alternate between two tasks that are usually otherwise performed singly. The best example of this is the Trail Making Test (Part B). The examinee is used to counting by 1's and reciting the alphabet, but on this task, the testee must alternate between connecting numbers to connecting letters scattered on a page. Thus, the subject connects 1 to A to 2 to B, etc. The set must be shifted from numbers to letters back to numbers. Input and output are discussed under "Alternating Attention". Another example is "knock, slap, chop" in which the subject sequentially performs these three movements repeatedly, shifting from knock to slap to chop and repeating the pattern. Input is audioverbal while output is motoric. On LNNB the examinee is asked to repetitively "show your teeth, stick out your tongue and place your tongue between your lower teeth and lower lip." Audioverbal input followed by visual input (demonstration) is paired with oral-motor output.

A third type of set shifting involves performing a familiar task in a novel way. That is, the individual must shift set from the usual expected response to a different response. This will be discussed under Novelty.

Novelty

Two set shifting tests that require novel responses are the Stroop Color Word Interference trial and the PASAT. The Interference trial of the Stroop presents color words (e.g., "red", "green") in a different color ink from the color word. The task is to rapidly name the color of the ink for the list of one hundred words and inhibit the customary response of reading the words. The PASAT requires the individual to shift from adding the number on the tape to the sum the examinee has just determined and named. Instead, the subject must add the new number to the last number heard on the tape before the examinee named out loud the sum of the previous two numbers. For example, if the numbers on the tape were 3, 8, 7, the subject would respond 11 (3+8), 15 (8+7). The temptation would be to give the second answer as "18" because the subject had just said "11" prior to hearing the next number "7". Input is visual for Stroop and output is verbal. For PASAT, input is auditory with verbal-numeric output.

Another type of novel task is one requiring the subject to generate responses according to a specific set of rules or constraints. The Ruff Figural Fluency Test is a good example. The individual has to draw nonsense designs that are different from each other and not like known designs. Input is verbal, output is motoric.

Problem Solving

This includes divergent and convergent thinking, inductive and deductive reasoning, planning ahead, and ability to draw inferences. Divergent and convergent thinking are inherent in Categories and Wisconsin Card Sort. The quantitative portion of the SILS and proverbs from the LNNB involve inductive reasoning while Block Design involves deductive reasoning. Tower of Hanoi and Porteus Mazes require planning ahead. Inferences are drawn from pictorial representations on Picture Arrangement from the WAIS III. Attention to subtle cues is necessary to determine the theme and correct sequence of the pictures to make a logical story. The LNNB picture sequences and picture description items involve inferential reasoning as well. Input is visual for all tests except LNNB proverbs, which has some auditory items as well as visual ones. Output is motoric for all but LNNB proverbs and picture descriptions, which are verbal.

Impulse Control

Perseveration is the most usual measure of impulsivity on neuropsychological tests. Categories and Wisconsin Card Sort have perseveration scores that reflect the degree to which the subject did not control the impulse to respond in the previously successful way that had now become incorrect or kept trying to use the same incorrect solution despite feedback that it was incorrect. Trails B and PASAT afford the opportunity to determine if and how often the individual failed to shift set and persisted in the overlearned pattern (e.g., 1 to 2 rather than 1 to A or A to B rather than A to 2 on Trails B; adding the new number to the previous sum rather than to the previously named number on the tape on PASAT). Number of perseverations is measured on alternating figures on the LNNB and Dementia Rating Scale (DRS). Bimanual motor alternation tasks can be examined for perseverations on LNNB and DRS. Tapping patterns that are limited to a set number can be examined for failure to stop at that number on LNNB. Perseverations and intrusions are identified on Auditory Consonant Trigrams and AVLT. Total number of perseverations on LNNB can be compared to a normative data set in the manual.

Categories, Card Sort, Trails B, PASAT, Trigrams and AVLT have been discussed previously and their input and output characteristics are also summarized in the Appendices. LNNB and DRS alternating figures have visual input and motoric output. LNNB tapping items have audiovisual input and motor output.

Judgment

Social judgment and ability to make reasonable decisions can be examined. Tests involving social judgment include Comprehension from WAIS III and IV and Picture Arrangement from WAIS III. The former is a verbal measure of knowledge of social expectations while the latter is a nonverbal measure applying social knowledge and judgment. The picture sequences on LNNB require knowledge and application of social situations and humor. Reasonable decisions are assessed on LNNB list-learning when the individual has to make an estimate of his next performance based on his previous one. Comprehension is presented in the audioverbal channel and output is verbal. Picture Arrangement has visual input and motor output. LNNB picture sequences are visually presented with motor output. Performance estimate on the LNNB word list involves audioverbal feedback as input and the verbal estimate as output.

Chapter 3
Treatment Strategies

Following brain injury there is an acute phase during which the brain undergoes reorganization and changes that permit it to recover from the initial effects of the injury. Most brain injuries lead to cognitive disruption but some or all of the functioning returns to normal by the end of the acute phase of mild traumatic brain injury (mTBI). For example, Alexander (1995) reports that the typical uncomplicated traumatic brain injury cases recover in 6–12 weeks and 85–90% of mild traumatic brain injury patients return to normal functioning within a year following injury. At 3 months post-injury "neurologic recovery is substantial" and most of these have shown significant improvement or recovery by 6–9 months post-injury. Kashluba et al. (2008) found that about 20% of 110 consecutively admitted patients reported persistent symptoms at 3 months post injury. The observation that at least 10% of mTBI patients have sequelae beyond the acute phase has been made in studies with large numbers of subjects [von Wild (2008) with 5,000 cases and Christensen et al. (2009) using a population-based cohort of 1.6 million individuals]. In a meta-analysis of 39 studies involving 1,463 cases of mild traumatic brain injured individuals and 1,191 controls, Vanderploeg et al. (2009) concluded that mTBI, "even in the chronic phase years post injury", is not benign and is associated with headaches, sleep problems and memory difficulties and can complicate or prolong recovery from other conditions. Belanger et al. (2005) found no residual neuropsychological impairment in unselected or prospective samples of mTBI patients, but they found that clinic-based samples had greater cognitive sequelae at 3 months or longer post injury. In another study (Vanderploeg et al. 2005) mTBI patients who had suffered their injuries an average of 8 years earlier were compared to matched control groups. While no significant differences were found across 15 measures on a standard neuropsychological battery, significant subtle differences were found in attention and working memory. All of these findings are consistent with the existence of a small subset of mTBI patients who do not make a full recovery following the acute phase. However, meta-analytic reviews have been cited as support for "no indication of permanent impairment on neuropsychological testing by 3 months" (McCrae 2007). The above summary suggests that this is an oversimplification and is not supported by

M. H. Podd, *Cognitive Remediation for Brain Injury and Neurological Illness*,
DOI: 10.1007/978-1-4614-1975-4_3, © Springer Science+Business Media, LLC 2012

the research, as subtle differences were found. The meta-analytic conclusions cited to suggest postacute effects of mTBI do not exist (e.g., Belanger et al. 2005; Frencham et al. 2005) have been criticized by Pertab et al. (2009) who reanalyzed the data from the Binder et al. (1997) meta-analysis and the Frencham et al. (2005) meta-analysis by recategorizing according to mechanism of injury, diagnostic criteria used, assessment tools used and whether symptomatic groups were considered separately. They demonstrated that clinically relevant information could be obscured by meta-analytic procedures that combined data that was methodologically and statistically heterogeneous. Clinically significant and lasting effects for a subset of neuropsychological measures were identified. In reviewing imaging and neuronal biomarker studies along with postmortem findings of patients with persistent post-concussive syndrome (symptoms persisting beyond 3 months postconcussion) Bigler (2008) concluded that there was "indisputable evidence that structural pathology can be present in mTBI". He also cites evidence that patients with persistent post-concussive syndrome show functional imaging deficits when the cognitive demand is increased although they did not show deficits at rest or while performing less demanding cognitive tasks. Using diffusion tensor imaging MacDonald et al. (2011) found that 6–12 months post injury 47 of 63 mTBI patients had abnormal brain scans consistent with evolving injuries.

Stroke patients frequently return to premorbid functioning within 3-to-6 months after the CVA and according to Wiederholt (1982) many make substantial improvement within 3–4 weeks. For this reason, testing during the acute phase is not necessarily useful for anything except documentation of deficits that may spontaneously recover. Cognitive remediation is not necessarily helpful during the acute phase of TBI or stroke as there is no way to clinically demonstrate that the intervention was superior to simply waiting. The next section will discuss the neurological mechanisms that could account for recovery during the acute phase. This will be followed by the intervention strategies that may enhance the likelihood of stimulating these mechanisms in the post-acute phase. The interventions have been demonstrated to produce behavioral change in the direction of improved cognitive functioning.

Mechanisms of Recovery

Diaschisis (Von Monakow 1914/1960) refers to the functional disturbance of brain regions distant from the actual site of injury during the acute phase. This is caused by metabolic and physiological changes and/or functional inhibition or deinhibition of areas distant to the injury site. These changes are usually temporary and the brain usually reverts to its normal functioning. Most mild closed head injuries recover completely because the cognitive disruption was largely due to these temporary, reversible effects. Bigler (2008) reports that much pathology of acute concussions is likely due to transient biochemical induced neurotransmitter disruption after which the brain usually returns to normal functioning. Povlishock and

Katz (2005) and Hall et al. (2005) report cytoskeletal disruptions occuring in the acute phase that make cells temporarily less functional.

Other mechanisms of recovery have been summarized in the literature (e.g., Almi and Finger 1992; Stein et al. 1995). Axonal regeneration refers to functional regrowth at the site of the axonal injury. Collateral sprouting may also occur following axonal injury. The area that has been damaged may no longer be functional, but connections may sprout from another part of the axon and function to pass information to neighboring cells in the brain.

Synaptic supersensitivity or denervation supersensitivity refers to reorganization at the synapse such that areas specialized to bind with certain chemicals become respecialized and provide additional binding sites for specific neurotransmitters. Information can thus be passed across the synapse even when less neurotransmitter is released because of the brain damage. The additional sites increase the likelihood that most of the limited amount of neurotransmitter released will find a binding site and pass the information.

Diaschisis is a phenomenon of the acute phase following brain injury as are biochemical induced neurotransmitter disruption and cytoskeletal disruption. Sprouting and synaptic supersensitivity may occur during the acute and possibly the postacute phase. It is in the postacute phase that cognitive remediation is indicated. After residual deficits have been identified and alternate functional systems have been constructed, treatment may proceed using compensatory strategy development. Following successful compensation, restitutional strategies may be undertaken in an effort to restore the original, premorbid functioning. The underlying neurological mechanisms for restitution have yet to be definitely identified but they may involve synaptic supersensitivity and/or sprouting that have been potentiated by the restorative strategies.

Compensatory Strategies

The development of compensatory strategies will be discussed in detail in the next chapter. Based upon the neuropsychological testing profile the patient's cognitive weaknesses can be treated by teaching him alternative strategies that rely upon his assessed strengths instead of the weaknesses. Thus, an individual with spatial memory problems can be taught to code information using the auditory-verbal channel or the visual–verbal channel, if these are relatively intact. Someone with impulse control problems can be taught to verbally talk his way through the situation instead of reacting first. This allows him to think and evaluate prior to responding.

The next chapter will describe the various compensatory mechanisms that can be taught on each of the exercises in NeurXercise. The development of compensatory mechanisms allows the individual to again perform adequately in the targeted domain. However, speed and efficiency are sometimes negatively impacted when the compensatory mechanism introduces several intervening steps in order to circumvent the damaged link in the functional chain. Because of this, it is worth considering the possibility of restoring the damaged functional system. This may be possible through the use of restitutional strategies.

Restitutional Strategies

The basic premise requires the therapist to take the previously described treatment process one step beyond compensation. After accomplishing an effective compensatory strategy within a specific domain, this strategy is then used as a basis to "rebuild" the old, dysfunctional system. That is, following the successful development of an alternate functional system, this method of compensation becomes the basis for creating a system that allows for redevelopment of the old functional system.

I will provide a few examples to help clarify how this is accomplished. A patient with an auditory verbal memory deficit is taught to use a visual imagery strategy to recall verbal material. When this is done successfully, the patient continues to do verbal memory exercises using the compensatory strategy, but gradually introduces the auditory verbal mode as well. That is, he/she says the word to be recalled in addition to making a visual image that will become a cue for the word. Increasingly, the recitation of the word is emphasized while the visualization is de-emphasized, tapered and eventually deleted from the memory process. The same process is used in reverse order if the patient has a visual memory deficit and has learned to compensate with verbal strategies. Patient report and observation of others helps document the extent to which the patient is performing at the premorbid level.

Visual–spatial deficits can be minimized by teaching executive strategies. For example, if tracking and aiming are problems on *Dartboard* (described in the next chapter), the patient can "solve the problem" and compensate by identifying the spot on the screen from which the dart should be thrown. Thus, the patient focuses on the spot and releases the dart when it comes into his view instead of tracking it. When this is well-established, the patient focuses slightly before this spot and tracks the briefest distance. Speed of the dart can also be slowed so that the task can more easily be accomplished. The amount of distance to be tracked can be increased gradually while the dart travels slowly and the required speed of tracking is slow. As the patient improves, speed of the dart can be increased gradually. In the final phase the patient is tracking and aiming at the normal speed with normal performance. The patient and others can report on real-life tracking and spatial functioning. Successful implementation of restitutional strategies will be exemplified in the NeurXercise Casebook section of this book.

The next chapter will provide a complete description of the cognitive remediation program, NeurXercise, and the various compensatory and learning mechanisms that can be utilized for effective treatment.

Chapter 4
Cognitive Remediation with NeurXercise

The Podd and Krehbiel study (2006) utilized the computer-assisted cognitive remediation software, NeurXercise (Podd and Seelig 1989, 1994). This software has been used successfully on post-acute patients with mild, mild/moderate and severe head injuries, strokes, cerebrovascular disease, temporal lobectomies, frontal resections, toxic exposure and subcortical disease (Podd et al. 1996; Podd 1998a, b, c, 2000; Podd and Seelig 1999). It was also shown to be efficacious in the treatment of children with severe emotional disturbance and concomitant attention deficit disorder (Garlaza et al. 1999). It has been used for compensation and restitution training, which was discussed in the last chapter. The present chapter presents a neuropsychological analysis of NeurXercise that parallels the format of Chap. 2, assessment in treatment planning, and conveniently allows for identification of exercises that will likely help in remediation based on the neuropsychological testing results. The salient input–output characteristics of the exercises are summarized in Appendices J through N.

NeurXercise is comprised of 30 multi-level game-like exercises falling into the domains of attention/concentration, visual perception/spatial skill, memory, reasoning, judgment and daily living skills. The NeurXercise manual (Podd and Seelig, 1994) identifies specific targets and the different exercises used to practice the skills. These targets include focused, sustained, alternating and divided attention, processing speed, visual-motor, visual-perceptual and visual spatial abilities, immediate and delayed verbal and nonverbal memory, facial memory, impulse control, abstract reasoning, and problem solving. The game-like exercises have adjustable parameters so that the exercises can be individualized to meet the level of ability at which the specific patient can function. Examples of this procedure will be presented in the casebook section of the book.

Once the treatment targets have been identified, several exercises are selected that focus on each target while containing elements of the patient's assessed neuropsychological strengths. For example, if visual tracking and visual-spatial skills are intact while attention is not, *Dartboard, Space Probe and Run Silent* would be good choices for attention training as they have the tracking and spatial components as part of the task. If a patient is assessed to have problems with

M. H. Podd, *Cognitive Remediation for Brain Injury and Neurological Illness*,
DOI: 10.1007/978-1-4614-1975-4_4, © Springer Science+Business Media, LLC 2012

visual-nonverbal memory while auditory-verbal memory is relatively intact, exercises and help screens are chosen that teach an auditory-verbal strategy on visual-nonverbal memory tasks. This allows the development of a compensatory mechanism to bypass the deficit by using other brain functions. The compensatory strategy is used on different exercises to increase the likelihood that the strategy is practiced and applied in different situations rather than the patient learning merely how to approach one situation without generalization to others. As the skill becomes more effective in producing "normal" scores on the exercises, the therapist discusses application to daily life and situations. The patient is encouraged to practice using the compensatory mechanism in these real life situations as well as continuing to practice their application on a variety of exercises provided for homework.

The remainder of this chapter will be devoted to discussion of different treatment targets and the specific exercises that can be harnessed to remediate function through the development of compensatory mechanisms and approaches aimed at restitution of function.

Attention and Concentration

Focused Attention

The most elementary level of attention is focused attention. It requires the patient to attend briefly to a stimulus and then respond. On a daily basis we are required to use focused attention when we respond to simple questions (e.g., how are you?, what's up?, what time will you get home?), fill out forms requiring basic demographic information (e.g., name, age, address), and put the groceries in the right place (e.g., the ice cream goes in the freezer not the cupboard). NeurXercise contains four verbal focused attention exercises and three nonverbal ones.

Get Q (Level 1) is a verbal focused attention task. It requires the respondent to press a key whenever a *Q* appears on screen. The appearance of letters is set at a random,variable ratio and the inter-stimulus interval is programmable by the trainer. Positive comments appear on the computer screen when the respondent is accurate, and factual or humorous feedback appears when errors occur. The trainer programs whether the trainee's reaction time appears following every *Q*. The goal is accurate responding at a speed comparable to that found among our unimpaired sample. Thereafter, one may wish to work toward premorbid level if the trainee functioned at a higher than average level. Input is visual-alphabetic and output is motoric.

Another verbal focused attention task in the NeurXercise software is *Type It*. It presents a simple instruction and allows the respondent to decide when he/she is ready to follow the single command. The respondent removes the command from the screen when he/she is ready and then follows the direction. On Level 1 the commands are very simple and exercise the most basic focused attention, e.g., "Type the number'1'." On Level 2 the instructions require one response with the right hand and a different one with the left, or verbal responses preceded or followed by manual ones. By Level 3 the trainee must perform mental operations on the focused attention task, e.g., "Type your age plus 100 and type three kinds of fruits." Input is visual-verbal while output is usually motoric.

Nonverbal focused attention is practiced on *Flasher*, an exercise that presents flashes of colored squares accompanied by a different tone and requires the trainee to repeat the tonal sequence by clicking on the correct sequence of squares immediately after hearing and seeing the stimulus. Parameters can be set to present a random sequence of tone-color squares drawn from 2, 3 or 4 different stimuli. Duration of the stimulus and choice of help screens are under the control of the trainer. Help screens are alternate functional systems, including use of the color name in lieu of the visual image of the color or the pitch of the tone, use of a numbering code for each square, use of a letter to stand for each square (e.g., R= red), or spatial recall in lieu of color or tone. Each strategy can be applied audi-overbally or visually, according to the trainer's recommendation based upon neuropsychological testing results. Input is visual and auditory; output is motoric.

Space Probe allows the trainee to release a rocket that travels vertically until it reaches a designated region, at which time the trainee clicks on a button to fire the rocket. Each trial is under the trainee's control and thus it is discrete and practices focused attention. The trainer sets the speed of the rocket and sound effects may be used to enhance motivation or disabled when they are felt to hamper function. Amount of external guidance in determining the center of the target differentiates the first from the second level. Input is visual and output is motoric.

Sustained Attention

Sustained attention involves ability to concentrate on a task continually, usually from less than a minute to several minutes or hours. Assessment measures of continuous performance tap sustained attention. Reading a novel, studying for an exam and attending to a movie all require sustained attention. There are six verbal sustained attention exercises and six nonverbal ones. The nonverbal sustained attention exercises are part of the Perception module and practice perceptual/spatial skill as well as sustained attention. These will be discussed under perception.

Get Q (Levels 2 and 3) require rapid responses to every stimulus that appears on screen. As with Level 1 there is a standard response when *Q* comes on screen. However, a different response is required when any other letter appears. Letters are presented at a variable ratio and the duration of the task (and thus sustained attention) is about five to seven minutes. Like Level 1, input is visual-alphabetic and output is motoric.

Two in One (Levels 1, 2, 3, 4) involves approximately one minute of sustained attention. The trainee must type alternating series of overlearned material on Levels 1 and 2, and perform an alternating series using a "serial threes paradigm" (i.e., adding three to each previous number and letter typed) on Levels 3 and 4. Level 2 has an added impulse control component that will be discussed under Judgment. On all levels input is visual-verbal (written instructions) and output is motoric (typing alpha-numeric sequences).

The nonverbal sustained attention exercises include *Run Silent* (Levels 1, 2, 3 and 4) and *Dartboard* (Levels 1 and 2). These will be discussed under the Perception section of this chapter.

Alternating Attention

Alternating attention requires the trainee to perform attentional shifts between two different tasks. Attention is focused on one task followed by complete shift to another task in alternating fashion. There is a sustained attentional factor built into these tasks whenever they take more than a few seconds to complete. A routine example might include beginning to write a paper for school, interrupting it to talk with someone about your plans for the evening, agreeing to call them back to continue the conversation, return to the paper for a while, shift back to the phone call, etc. There are six verbal alternating attention exercises and two nonverbal exercises.

The verbal alternating attention tasks are *Get Q* (Levels 2 and 3) and *Two in One* (Levels 1–4). The trainee must make different responses depending upon the specific stimulus that appears on screen during *Get Q*. All levels of *Two in One* require alternating between numbers and letters. *Run Silent* (Levels 3 and 4) are the nonverbal alternating attention tasks. This will be discussed in the Perception section.

Divided Attention

In contrast to alternating attention, divided attention requires the performance of two or more tasks simultaneously rather than sequentially. It is commonly referred to as multi-tasking. Examples in daily life include talking on the phone while working on the computer, watching TV and holding a conversation, listening to phone messages while reading the newspaper, and holding two or more conversations simultaneously (e.g., answering one person while listening to the statements of another and then responding to that person). There are two divided attention exercises on the software. One of the exercises presents two homogeneous tasks (both visual) and the other utilizes heterogeneous ones (one task is visual and the other is auditory). Sustained attention is an inherent part of divided attention. On the exercises below, alternating attention is also incorporated into the divided attention tasks.

Double Trouble (Level 1) combines *Get Q* and *Space Probe*. The rocket drops rapidly and continuously and the trainee must click on the FIRE button with the mouse when the probe is within the target range, thus practicing visual-nonverbal sustained attention. At the same time letters appear on screen and the trainee must press the ENTER key for *Qs* and the space bar for all other letters. This aspect of the task incorporates alternating attention. *Get Q* provides visual-verbal input and *Space Probe* presents visual-nonverbal input. Both tasks require motor output and must be performed simultaneously, practicing divided attention.

Double Trouble (Level 2) presents the trainee with pairs of tones while he/she is engaged in *Space Probe*. *Space Probe* is presented identically on Level 1 and Level 2. The tones are drawn from the four standard tones used in *Flasher*. The trainee presses the ENTER key if the tones are identical and the space bar if they are not. This aspect of the task incorporates alternating attention. Both exercises (*Space Probe* and *Flasher's* tones) have a motor output but there is an auditory input from the tones as opposed to the visual input on *Space Probe*. Both exercises are performed simultaneously.

Processing Speed

The rate at which the brain takes in and reacts to information is called processing speed. Reaction time is sometimes used as an indicator. Evoked potential is a neurological test that directly measures this variable that is frequently impacted by brain injury. Ecologically, we observe if someone is "quick on the uptake", responds quickly and even anticipatorily to situations, or can quickly balance a checkbook. There are seven verbal processing speed exercises and seven nonverbal ones.

The three levels of *Get Q* record reaction time, which is a reflection of processing speed. The accuracy of the trainee's response is important in determining if the speed was due to rapid processing or impulsive reactivity. The scores in the patient's file identify accurate and inaccurate responses and the associated response speeds. All four levels of *Two in One* provide a time to completion score as well as number of errors. Processing speed is reflected in time to completion, as the exercise does not terminate until correct responses have been given, analogous to Trail Making. These constitute the verbal processing speed exercises.

Dartboard (Levels 1 and 2), when set to rapid speeds, requires quick processing. This exercise will be discussed under the perception section. *Invaders* can be set at three levels of difficulty, requiring increasingly rapid processing. This exercise will also be discussed in detail under the perception section. *Run Silent* (Levels 1 and 2) can program the ship and the plane to travel at faster speeds and thereby create enhanced demands on nonverbal processing speed. This exercise will be discussed under the perception section.

Perception

Visual Scanning and Tracking

Attending to visual movements, spatial location, and visual shifts involves visual scanning and tracking. It is a major element on the Trail Making Test. It is an element of routine eye examinations. In everyday life we track people walking or running, we scan a book or newspaper, or keep an eye on a suspicious character. There are three verbal exercises that include a scanning/tracking element and 12 nonverbal ones. Input is always visual and output is always motoric on these exercises.

The letters appear in random sectors of the computer screen on *Get Q* (Levels 1–3). This builds in a scanning requirement for these verbal exercises. If the individual does not scan the screen efficiently, response time will be negatively impacted.

Both levels of *Space Probe* require the trainee to track the rocket until it reaches the target range. Similarly, both levels of *Dartboard* place the same demand on the respondent. Darts spontaneously and continuously run across the bottom of the screen and must be tracked until they reach the target area when the trainee "throws" them up to the target. The score is determined on closeness to the bullseye.

Tracking and scanning are required on the four levels of *Run Silent*. The trainee fires a rocket from a moving ship toward a moving plane on Level 1, requiring scanning and tracking of both transports. On Level 2 the moving plane drops a bomb on the moving ship, with the same scanning and tracking requirements as Level 1. Levels 3 and 4 require the trainee to alternate Level 1 and 2 tasks.

Invaders from the Fifth Dimension may be set at three increasingly rapid speeds. The trainee tracks the movement of the missile, changes its direction to move to an intercept course, and redirects it when the invader jumps to a different place on the screen. On *Bomber* a plane is tracked and bombs released to hit a target that is large at first but becomes increasingly small as the trainee is successful.

Spatial Organization

This refers to orientation in space. It is reflected in ability to align the grooves in Grooved Pegboard, correctly orienting the blocks for placement on Tactile Performance Test, and proper placement of the hands on clock drawings. In daily function it is encountered in sense of direction, telling time (on nondigital time pieces), and many home improvement projects. There are 20 nonverbal exercises and four verbal exercises that include a spatial component.

Each level of *Flasher* has an increasing spatial component (stimuli appear in two locations in space on Level 1 through four locations in space on Level 3). Assessment of distance and trajectory for intercept are spatial components on all four levels of *Run Silent*. Level 4 presents ships and planes at different heights and depths during each successive trial, requiring continuous recalculation of the spatial parameters necessary for interception. Thus, Level 4 has the most demand on spatial abilities among the four levels.

Invaders requires movement and changes in direction through space within the restriction of moving only at right angles. This is true regardless of the level practiced, as level variation is based on increased demand for speed of response without changes in spatial requirements. *Bomber* requires spatial skill toward the end of the exercise when only a few small targets are on screen and the plane has to drop a bomb directly on these targets.

All three levels of *Strategy* involve a multi-level tic-tac-toe game with success defined as a sequence of four in a spatial pattern. This will be discussed more fully under the Reasoning section of Executive Functions. *Hid in the Grid* requires spatial computation in trying to find a target hidden within a grid. This exercise will be discussed under the Judgment section of Executive Functions.

Concentration requires spatial memory on both levels and will be discussed under the Memory section. *Towers of Hanoi* is an exercise in spatial problem solving and will be discussed under Reasoning in the Executive Functions domain. *Map Reading* (Levels 1 and 2) involves spatial negotiation to travel from one point to another and will be discussed under Daily Living Skills. *Detective* (Level 1) includes spatial orientation as one of the principles in this problem solving exercise that is discussed under the Reasoning section of Executive Functions.

Under verbal spatial orientation exercises is *Golf*. The trainee gets verbal feedback about distance traveled and distance required to reach the hole in the effort to sink the ball. This is discussed in more detail under the Judgment section of Executive Functions. *Two in One* (Levels 3 and 4) from the Attention module requires mental addition, which has a component of carrying over in space when it reaches two digits (e.g., 19+3 requires spatial carryover from the tens column to the units column). *Detective* (Level 2) is a verbal problem solving exercise that includes a spatial principle (palindromes). This exercise is discussed in the Reasoning section of Executive Functions.

Memory

Verbal Memory

There are six verbal memory exercises. *Memory Game* involves recalling letter strings on Level 1 and increasingly long strings of words on Level 2. As the subject sees more lists of words and the words become more similar (e.g., baseball and basketball, hat and cap), an interference factor is introduced. Trainees are taught to code the letters into nonsense words on Level 1 and into a story or visual image on Level 2. This has everyday application to coding and recall of verbal material, e.g., items to get from the store or names of recording artists, such as Mobey Grape or Ice T. Input is visual-verbal and output is motoric.

Foreign Intrigue involves recognition of letters on Level 2 and words on Level 3. Thus, both levels present visual-verbal input and motor output. *Shopping List* is based on the same paradigm and literature that the CVLT drew upon. In fact, this exercise was actually developed independent of the CVLT and before it was published. It will be discussed in detail under the Daily Living section. *Buying Power* (Level 3) requires the trainee to recall the prices of goods and services learned on Level 2. This is discussed in more detail in the Daily Living section.

Visual Nonverbal Memory

There are 13 visual nonverbal exercises, requiring recall and recognition of objects, position in space, symbols and faces. The three levels of *Flasher* have been discussed under Focused Attention. *Concentration* requires the trainee to find and match objects hidden behind doors on Level 1. Level 2 uses faces on the same task. Help screens that can be selected by the therapist include audio-overbal coding, spatial coding, and systematic organizational responding. The task presents visual input with motor output. *Symbol Memory* involves free recall and cued recall for a series of symbols of increasing length that appear on the screen for a brief time. The symbols are readily codable into words so that audioverbal compensatory strategies may be applied. The exercise involves visual input and motor output.

Line Up is a matching to sample exercise on Level 1. The trainee sees a face for a brief exposure (time is programmable by therapist). This is followed by a brief delay (again programmable by therapist), and then there is a "line up" of four faces (the target and three foils). The trainee clicks the mouse on the "guilty party". Positive feedback appears on screen for correct responses and comical (e.g., "that's the police chief") or factual (e.g., "No") feedback appear for incorrect responses. Toward the end of the exercise the foils are the same face with minor differences (e.g., no tie, smile, head tilt difference).

Line Up (Level 2) is a matching to nonsample paradigm. Four faces of "criminals" are presented sequentially and then a "line up" appears. The task is to click the mouse on the "innocent party" who did not appear previously. Feedback is as above. *Line Up* (Level 3) follows the format and instructions of Level 1 but the target is a different pose from the initial stimulus (e.g., different clothes, different lighting, several years before or after the original pose). On all levels input is visual and output is motoric.

Foreign Intrigue involves facial recognition on Level 1. Thus, input is visual and output motoric. *Time Travel* requires long-term facial memory. Famous faces appear from each decade dating back to the 1940s. On Level 1 the trainee must recognize the name of the target from a list of choices. On Level 2 the trainee must recall and type the name of the famous individual. Thus, Level 1 provides visual-facial and visual-verbal input while Level 2 provides only visual- facial input. Output is motoric on both levels.

Facial Memory

There are eight facial memory exercises. *What's My Name* is discussed in detail under Daily Living Skills. It requires the subject to recognize a face and pair it with a name. All three levels of *Line Up* involve facial recognition, as does *Concentration* (Level 2). *Time Travel* requires recognition of famous faces on Level 1 and recall of the names of those people on Level 2. *Detective* (Level 1), discussed under the Reasoning section of Executive Functions, includes recognition of famous faces in order to correctly draw some of the analogies.

Delayed Memory

There are six exercises for delayed memory. *Concentration* (Levels 1 and 2) allows the trainee to repeat the same configuration he/she has just completed, thus allowing for evaluation of learning and delayed recall of the information previously presented. The therapist can lengthen the stimulus–response delay interval on *Line Up* (Levels 1, 2 and 3), thus introducing various levels of delayed memory. *Time Travel* involves long-term memory, with delays spanning decades.

Method of Access

There are 11 exercises that use free recall. These are *Memory Game* (Levels 1 and 2), *Shopping List*, *Buying Power* (Level 3), *What's My Name*, *Time Travel* (Level 2), and all levels of *Flasher* and *Concentration*. Recognition is involved in eight exercises. It is practiced on all levels of *Line Up* and *Foreign Intrigue*, Level 1 of *Detective* and *Time Travel* (Level 1). *Symbol Memory* allows for free recall and/or cued recall, as the symbols from which the string is chosen are on the screen and can serve as cues.

Executive Functions

Set Shifting

This is an executive function in which the subject must switch to a new or different behavior from a previously learned behavior or one in which he/she is currently engaged. Seven set shifting exercises are described under "Alternating Attention". In addition, there are six other exercises that include this executive function. *Mission Decode* requires set shifting several times during each level of the exercise, as the principle upon which the correct answer is based changes from time to time. The same is true for both levels of *Detective*. Input is visual and output motoric for all levels of both exercises. Both levels of *Double Trouble* require different responses to the stimuli that are presented and thus require the trainee to shift set momentarily in order to make the proper response to each stimulus.

Problem Solving: Reasoning and Convergent/Divergent Thinking

The are 10 exercises requiring divergent and convergent thinking, relevant to cognitive flexibility. All three levels of *Vocabulary* involve convergent thinking and deductive reasoning. The trainee is given several clues upon which to base a guess as to the word on the "wanted poster". With each failure an additional clue is provided. All information should be utilized to increase the likelihood that the correct word will be chosen. The words and the clues become more difficult as the levels increase. Input is visual-verbal and output is motoric (typing the guessed word). *Detective* (Level 1) is a pictorial analogy exercise, the basis of which shifts without warning. The trainee must flexibly evaluate the feedback and develop a new strategy that works (divergent thinking). That is, the trainee must generate alternate principles upon which the analogies are based. This requirement occurs several times during the exercise. Input is visual; output is motoric. On Level 2 the requirement is the same but the stimuli are words instead of pictures (visual-verbal input with motor output). On Levels 2 and 3 of *Strategy* the trainee must pay attention to the computer's strategy and potential to win as well as pursuing his/her own strategy. On the first level the computer responds randomly and therefore this level does not present a challenge to cognitive flexibility. On Level 2 the computer plays defensively while on Level 3 it uses offensive and defensive strategies. Thus, on Level 3 the trainee must generate a strategic plan (reasoning) and flexibly shift when the computer's moves disrupt the plan. On all levels input is visual and output is motoric.

Mission Decode is a two level exercise that involves concept formation (reasoning) and ability to flexibly shift one's conceptual thinking. The trainee must code the stimulus on the screen with one of four codes. The basis of the concept changes without warning and the patient must flexibly shift to generate another concept that again will produce correct responses. Every miss moves a bomb one step closer to detonation. Level 2 includes more difficult concepts than Level 1. *Spies* also involves unannounced shifts in concept upon which the correct answer is based. The stimuli are four faces and the "spy" or person who is different from the others must be selected based on concepts that are at times abstract and at times concrete. This involves a reasoning process. Input is visual and output motoric on both *Mission Decode* and *Spies*.

Problem Solving: Planning Ahead

There are 12 exercises that include a component of foresight for effective performance. *Strategy* is a multi-dimensional tic-tac-toe game against the computer. As previously discussed, the trainee must plan a strategy to win on all three levels and anticipate the computer's strategy on Level 3. *Invaders*, discussed under perception, requires the trainee to formulate a strategic approach and be ready to change course if the invader "makes a jump through hyperspace" to a different location on the screen. *Map Reading* (Levels 1 and 2) requires the trainee to plan the shortest route to a destination. It is discussed under Daily Living.

Body Language (Level 2) requires the trainee to anticipate the consequences of different actions based upon cues from the target pictures (e.g., facial expressions, muscular tension, body posture). Input is visual while output is motoric. On Level 3 of *Run Silent*, discussed under perception, the trainee must plan for the proper trajectory, depending upon whether it is time to fire the rocket or drop the bomb. *Towers of Hanoi* is a classic executive function task requiring planning and foresight to move discs from one peg to another within prescribed constraints. Specifically, four discs are arranged from largest to smallest on a peg and have to be moved such that they are in the same order on a different peg. However, larger pegs can not be placed on top of smaller pegs. The number of moves to reach the correct solution is automatically recorded in the patient's file. Success requires advanced planning so that each move should be made based on anticipating how this will meet the goal in the shortest number of moves.

Number Guesser (Levels 1 and 2) requires the trainee to use feedback from his/her guesses to plan the next "guess." On Level 1 the patient has to guess a number between 1 and 100 and is given feedback using a revised range following the guess (e.g., if the guess is "17" and the target is "50" then the new feedback is that the number is "too small", suggesting the target lies between "18 and 100"). On Level 2 the trainee has to guess a four-digit number and is provided feedback as to how many digits were in the "secret number" and how many were in the correct position. The number of guesses to reach the correct answer is automatically recorded in the patient's file. Input is visual and output is motor-numeric. *Hid in the Grid* is a spatial analog to *Number Guesser*. The trainee clicks the mouse on a square within a grid and receives feedback as to direction in which the hidden object lies. The objective is to find the hidden object in as few guesses as possible. Input is visual and output is motoric.

Impulse Control

There are 23 exercises with an impulse control element. Both levels of *Mission Decode* and *Detective* require set shifting and avoidance of perseveration. Both levels of *Space Probe*, described under Focused Attention, require the trainee to wait while the rocket slowly descends. The trainee must not fire until the rocket comes into the target range. On *Get Q* (Level 1), described under Attention, the trainee must press a key when a Q appears but not when other letters appear on screen. On Levels 2 and 3 the trainee must avoid the impulse to press the more frequently correct key when the less frequently appearing target comes on screen. *Two in One* requires overcoming the impulse to follow numbers with numbers and letters with letters. On Level 2 there is a shift from two single digit-two single letters repeated (e.g., 11AA22BB) to two double digit-two single letters repeated (e.g., 1010JJ1111KK). The impulse is to continue to type as many key strokes for numbers as letters when the requirement is to shift from that set. This may result in typing "10JJ" instead of "1010JJ".

On *Invaders,* discussed under perception, the trainee must inhibit the impulse to continue the planned approach to the target when the invader "jumps" and "leaves behind a space mine" in the area previously occupied. Speed increases on each of the three levels of *Invaders*, jumps increase at each level and rapid responding and increased impulse control are required as the level increases.

On *Run Silent* (Levels 1, 2, 3 and 4), presented in perception, the trainee must wait for the craft and its target to be properly aligned before firing. On Levels 3 and 4 the trainee must not give into the impulse to use the same alignment plan for firing as was immediately used as the plan must alternate between different trajectories.

Body Language (Level 2) requires the trainee to carefully study all aspects of the pictured individual before making a decision about how to proceed with interpersonal interaction. Impulse control must be exercised if the patient is to avoid making a *social faux pas* and causing problems for himself or the other person. All three levels of *Vocabulary* require the trainee to guess a target word based on clues. No guess should fail to meet all of the conditions set forth in the clues. Such a failure would be suggestive of impulsivity.

Judgment

There are two social judgment exercises that require reading emotions. Based on facial expression, muscle tension and body posture, the patient must select which of two emotions are being portrayed on screen when practicing *Body Language*

(Level 1). On Level 2 the same evaluation of the affect portrayed is used as a basis for decision-making. Feedback identifies some of the likely consequences for the action chosen. Input is visual and output is motoric on both levels.

There are eight additional exercises that involve good judgment for decision making. Hypothesis testing is practiced on all levels of *Vocabulary, Mission Decode, Detective* and *Spies.*

Daily Living Skills

Skills that are encountered in daily life are the subject addressed in these exercises. Neuropsychologically, they are comprised of a combination of the skills already described above. There are nine exercises in this module. *Body Language* (Level 1) teaches identification of emotional states through depicting facial and tensional cues in the photographs presented. Level 2 requires the subject to draw inferences and make decisions based upon the assessment of the emotional state of the depicted individual. The ability to size up a social situation and make decisions based upon this information is critical to social and occupational functioning.

Buying Power (Level 1) provides relearning of monetary denomination relationships for those who have had this knowledge disrupted. Level 2 teaches the cost of goods and services, which is essential in encountering the world. Level 3 requires the subject to recall the cost of goods and services and calculate how much change they would receive if they paid X amount of dollars.

What's My Name teaches the peg-word system. Associations are learned to common names and this is generalized to generating associations to any names. The subject then sees faces and learns the name through visual association. For example, if the association is "Sue-shoe", then when a face is named "Sue", the trainee might picture a shoe on her ear and recall this "silly" image when he again sees the face. The trainee then decodes the recalled image of a "shoe on her ear" and remembers her name is "Sue." Remembering people's names is an invaluable skill in social and occupational situations. The peg-word technique has been used successfully by memory experts for many years.

Shopping List teaches different strategies for recalling lists of items or lists of companies. Strategies include categorization and alphabetical arrangement. This is helpful when an individual has to recall a number of related or unrelated items and will not be able to easily refer to a written list at the time that he/she is required to produce the information.

Map Reading involves ability to "drive" from one spot on a map to a target elsewhere on the map. Direction and "sharpness" of the turn are involved. Planning the shortest route and executing that plan are also aspects of the exercise. Level 2 is a more complex route than Level 1.

After the treatment plan has been carried out, it is necessary to determine the extent to which it has been successful. This is the topic of the next chapter.

Chapter 5
Treatment Generalization and Ecological Validity

There are several different levels at which the efficacy of treatment can be evaluated. If treatment is effective, we should be able to demonstrate it on many of these. At the most concrete level we should be able to demonstrate that patients improve on cognitive remediation tasks that were performed in the abnormal range at baseline. Secondly, they should improve beyond chance level on neuropsychological tests in the areas treated. Neurological measures should be examined for improved neurophysiological functioning following treatment. Finally, and most importantly, behavioral change should be demonstrated in the patient's daily functioning. Each of these methods will be examined and discussed in detail.

Performance on the Training Tasks

Tasks selected from NeurXercise for the treatment plan are those that fall outside of normal limits at baseline. Expected performance is covered in the NeurXercise manual (Podd and Seelig 1994) and updated data sets on selected exercises gathered in 1999 and 2005–2006. The computerized cognitive remediation program allows the trainer to track progress and demonstrate to the trainee and others the patient's steady progress and eventual accomplishment of the goal on each exercise. This can be conveniently graphed using the data that is automatically saved in the patient's file.

For each target within each cognitive domain in the treatment plan the same procedure may be followed. First, track the level and speed of improvement and demonstrate that the preset goal has been reached. For example, it may take 12 trials on *Get Q* (Level 1) for the patient to score a median speed below 6 seconds. On Level 2, which is more complicated, reaching this criterion for both Q's and not Q's in 10 trials would suggest generalization from Level 1 and improved performance on the more difficult task.

M. H. Podd, *Cognitive Remediation for Brain Injury and Neurological Illness*,   39
DOI: 10.1007/978-1-4614-1975-4_5, © Springer Science+Business Media, LLC 2012

After examining generalization within the levels of the exercise, look to generalization between the exercises. Initially, look to other exercises within the same target. For example, visual attention exercises or sustained attention ones should take less time to complete as others have been successfully performed. A Planning Ahead exercise like *Number Guesser* (Level 1), which teaches an optimizing strategy, should generalize to a similar exercise like *Hid in the Grid* and lead to more rapid accomplishment of the goal than was the case on *Number Guesser*. Further, the improvement in the skill should generalize such that exercises in other domains that include the trained skill will also improve more quickly. For example, successful set shifting on the attention task *Two in One* and the perception task *Run Silent* (Level 3) should lead to more efficient performance on the executive tasks that involve set shifting, e.g., *Mission Decode*, *Detective*.

Changes on Re-testing

The pre-set criteria for each exercise in the treatment plan are determined by either the normative data provided with NeurXercise, the performance recommended in the NeurXercise manual, or individualized criteria for patients whose premorbid functioning was lower or higher than "normal". When all criteria have been met or the therapist feels that the patient is incapable of improving further, the neuropsychological testing battery should be repeated. Scores that improve by a standard deviation or more can be appropriately considered "true" change rather than random fluctuation. Alternate forms of tests are preferable, when available. Some tests have norms for first and second test administrations on the same form and these norms are recommended for use when possible (e.g., Stuss et al., 1987). In the LNNB manual Table 14 presents the T score changes from baseline that represent significant differences at the 0.10, 0.05, and 0.01 levels for clinical scales, summary scales, factor scales, localization scales, and lateralization scales.

Examine statistically significant changes from baseline to post-treatment testing. Since the instruments used are sensitive to the cognitive skills that were identified in the treatment plan, improvement should reflect enhanced cognitive functioning in the target areas. The more tests that show improvement within a specific domain, the more likely the results are reflecting improved cognitive functioning. There should be little improvement in areas that were not treated unless the cause of the dysfunction was a cognitive area treated rather than the apparent cause of the deficit. For example, receptive language performance could improve dramatically following attention training if the language difficulty was actually due to distractibility. However, if due to true receptive language problems that were not addressed in treatment, this would be an area expected to be relatively unchanged on repeat testing. To the extent that this is so, it provides further evidence that positive change occurs in target areas but not in those areas that were untreated. This is the premise behind the multiple baseline method described by Golden et al. (1983).

There should be periodic follow-up testing to demonstrate that improvement has been maintained. While most studies that address maintenance of treatment effects look at a brief period of time, it is more persuasive to demonstrate stability or continued improvement over 2 to 5 years posttreatment. Since patients should be beginning treatment in the postacute phase after they and their doctors fail to see any further improvements, patient and physicians are impressed to see stable change and often continuing improvement, even after treatment has been terminated. It often follows that once the recovery process gets restarted with treatment, the patient continues to recover beyond the treatment span.

Neurophysiological Change

Working with the patient's neurologist can be very helpful in that neurological tests can be given periodically as well as neuropsychological tests. Patients with focused attention problems, as is frequently found in postconcussion syndrome, might have abnormal P300 readings on the evoked potential. Remediation might return these tracings to normal levels, demonstrating brain recovery through cognitive remediation. Electroencephalography (e.g., QEEG) can also help track neurophysiological changes.

Functional neuroimaging is another neurological tool that can be helpful in evaluating cognitive remediation. Correlation between cognitive deficits and abnormal imaging on PET, SPECT, or functional MRI can be examined. The neuroimaging can constitute a pretreatment baseline against which to measure changes following treatment. Changes at posttreatment can reflect neurological improvement. Functional neuroimaging also opens extremely exciting possibilities, such as identifying the neurological regions involved in the compensatory systems that have been developed during the course of cognitive remediation or the degree to which there is restoration of the old functional system when restitution was a treatment goal.

Ecological Validity

The most important factor in determining the efficacy of cognitive remediation is behavioral improvement in daily living functions. Work and school are important areas frequently impacted by brain damage. These should be carefully examined before treatment occurs and following the intervention. If the individual was unable to return to his/her occupation before treatment commenced, the intervention might target return to work and track progress on the job when the patient is able to return to the work force. The same is true if the patient had been a student prior to injury or wishes to return to school to retrain in a new occupation. Approaches to measuring work and school performance will be demonstrated in the NeurXercise casebook section of this volume.

Other major daily living skills that often prove problematic for brain injury patients center around interpersonal relationships. Examining changes in how the patient relates to his family, friends, and colleagues at work may be extremely important. Patients often feel "less than the person they were" and withdraw or become hostile and irritable, disrupting their interpersonal relationships. Improvement on cognitive skills will often lead to a more positive self-image and positive changes in relating. Supportive psychotherapy can also help the patient learn how to improve and recover from these disruptions with the individuals in their lives.

Patients may also experience shifts from premorbid activity in the spiritual arena. Anger at God or doubting their former religious beliefs because they feel they did not deserve to suffer cognitive and emotional disruption, could lead them to withdraw from a significant source of comfort and support. Again, it can be very helpful to talk with a therapist about the spiritual concerns.

Hobbies are another source of gratification that could be impacted as the brain damaged individual withdraws from his/her former life. If the brain dysfunction directly impacts ability to pursue the hobby, the treatment should target skills that will allow return to the hobby to at least some degree. If the problem is more psychological, then psychotherapy in conjunction with observable improvement should help.

Chapter 6
A NeurXercise Casebook

The advantages of using case material as well as group research data have been discussed by Golden et al. (1983) and Heilman (2002; Greiffenstein's review and discussion of Heilman's book, 2003). Golden et al. propose a multiple baseline approach to evaluating cases and demonstrating validity of treatment. The validity is reflected in improvements in treated areas, whereas no improvements are expected in untreated areas across multiple assessments. Heilman gives details of cases that are instructive and indicative of the major elements of the disorders studied. Earlier in this book I proposed a model that allows for multiple levels of evaluation of treatment efficacy. The multiple baseline approach fits well with this model. It also helps us to see the many subtle differences that exist among patients within a general diagnostic group as well as highlighting the major elements of the disorder as suggested by Heilman.

This chapter will present cases paralleling the approach presented in the earlier chapters. The clinical circumstances and picture will be presented followed by neuropsychological testing. The results of the testing will be the basis for treatment planning. The exercises will be identified and baselines established to determine which would be most helpful to the treatment. Progress on the exercises will be presented followed by posttreatment testing for assessing neuropsychological test changes.

Neurological test results will be examined when available. Finally, ecological validity and generalization will be assessed through examination of changes in patient symptoms, occupational functioning, social interaction, progress in medical compliance, etc. Following Heilman, a brief summary of what the cases illustrate about the specific problems will be presented.

Graphic illustrations of data on many of the cases discussed herein are posted on Springer's free online resource at http://extras.springer.com. I have chosen to include illustrations in the book that highlight different exercises, different levels of the exercises, ways to organize the data for graphic presentation, types of graphic presentation, multiple criteria for success, alternative compensatory and restorative strategies, and multiple testing measures for assessing pretreatment and

M. H. Podd, *Cognitive Remediation for Brain Injury and Neurological Illness*,
DOI: 10.1007/978-1-4614-1975-4_6, © Springer Science+Business Media, LLC 2012

posttreatment performance. The extra.spinger.com site contains similar graphic illustrations for the patients when the data sources are similar to those in the book.

I have organized this chapter of the book to try to be most helpful to the clinician. As such, cases in the first section are organized by etiology. This includes head trauma, blast injury, stroke, neurosurgical intervention (e.g., tumor resection, lobectomy), subcortical disorders, co-morbid conditions, attention deficit disorder, and learning disability. Symptoms and their remediation are described for each etiology. Typically, patients were seen for weekly sessions with homework assignments between sessions. In cases where multiple domains were impaired, each domain was treated to the criterion before treatment in the next domain was undertaken.

The next section covers remediation of specific cognitive domains. Thus, cases will focus on assessment and remediation of either attention, executive functioning or memory. Finally, cases will be presented that focus on the subpopulation of patients who are referred for treatment, e.g., geriatrics, litigants.

Etiology

Head Trauma

AF was a college sophomore when she was involved in a serious automobile accident. She was in a coma for 3 months. Neuroimaging revealed bifrontal hemorrhage and shearing, left parieto-occipital subdural hematoma, right subadrenal hematoma, frontal lobe punctate lesions, and lesions of the right pons. She completed inpatient rehabilitation and was discharged as having gained maximum medical benefit. She then entered a day treatment program for brain-injured patients and was later discharged as having received maximum benefit. She was still not satisfied with her level of recovery and entered another day treatment program. She made further gains and was discharged when they felt she could improve no further. About 3 years post injury she sought admission to a vocational rehabilitation project but she was rejected as too low functioning to benefit from the program. Three-and-a half years post injury, at age 23, she sought outpatient cognitive remediation. Testing with the LNNB revealed moderate to severe brain impairment with arrested compensation. Attention, memory, and reasoning were impaired and targeted for treatment. Arithmetic and motor skills were also impaired but not targeted for treatment as they were of less concern to the patient. Speech was impaired and being treated independently with speech therapy.

The following made up the NeurXercise treatment program. Alternating and sustained visual attention exercises included *Two in One* at Levels 1, 2, and 3. Because of her motor problems, only accuracy was targeted and not speed. Focused visual attention was practiced on *Run Silent* by having her focus on one spot and count from 1 to 9 before firing, rather than aiming and visually tracking. Another focused visual attention exercise was *Dartboard*, which was performed by

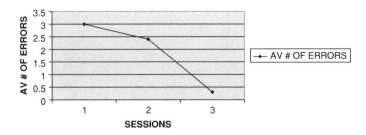

Fig. 6.1 AF alternating and sustained attention: accuracy on 2 in 1 (level 1)

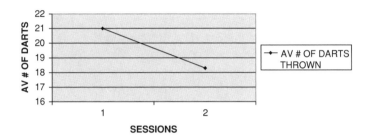

Fig. 6.2 AF focused attention: Dartboard 1 (500 pts)

looking at a specific spot and throwing the dart when it arrived at the spot (instead of tracking it to the spot, which would involve visual perception). Memory exercises included *Memory Game* 2, *Shopping List*, and *Concentration*. Executive functions were practiced on *Run Silent* 3, *Number Guesser* 2, *Hid in the Grid*, *Buying Power*, *Spies*, *Mission Decode*, *Detective*, and *Vocabulary*.

Figure 6.1 shows that sustained and alternating attention improved from a baseline of three errors to an average of 0.3 errors over two practice sessions beyond the baseline measure. The baseline was a single measure while the next two sessions comprised approximately ten measures each. She was able to perform without error on three consecutive trials during the last session and thereby met the criterion for completion of the exercise. On Level 2 there were only two of eight trials on which she made non-ataxic errors, i.e., she committed no attentional errors on the exercise during six of the eight times it was practiced. On Level 3 she made no errors on seven of eight practice runs. Using counting as opposed to the tracking strategy, she was able to make no more than one error half of the time she practiced *Run Silent* Level 1. On only four of 17 practice runs did she make more than two errors (baseline, with tracking, was 53 errors). Focused attention on *Dartboard* 1 improved over two sessions (see Fig. 6.2). The version used was an earlier version of the one currently in use and the number of points was apportioned somewhat differently. On Level 2 she likewise showed dramatic improvement over two sessions (see Fig. 6.3). Session 1 represents the baseline score, session 2 is her homework score, and session 3 is the score she received while working in front of the examiner.

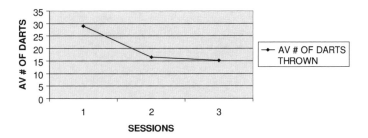

Fig. 6.3 AF focused attention: Dartboard 2 (500 pts)

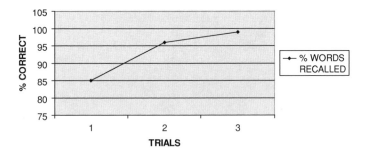

Fig. 6.4 AF list recall: Memory Game 2

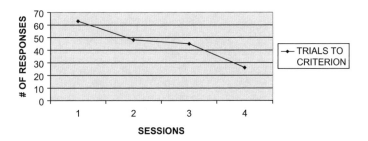

Fig. 6.5 AF spatial–nonverbal memory: Concentration

List recall was practiced on *Memory Game* 2 and S*hopping List*. Figure 6.4 shows that she recalled 85% of the words at baseline on *Memory Game* 2 and improved to 99% by the third attempt. At baseline, she required two attempts at each list contained on *Shopping List*. However, 9 months later, after practicing list learning strategies on *Memory Game* 2, she recalled all lists on the first exposure. On *Concentration* her first two sessions employed visual strategies and she took more than the targeted number of trials (below 30) to make all matches. Thereafter, she named the items aloud and made significant progress by using this auditory-verbal strategy (see Fig. 6.5), reaching the criterion for success by the second session on which she practiced the new strategy.

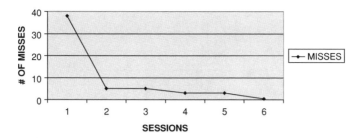

Fig. 6.6 AF executive functions: set shifting on Run Silent 3

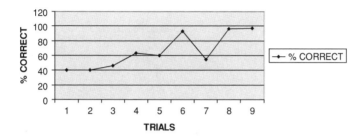

Fig. 6.7 AF executive functions: set shifting and reasoning on Mission Decode

The executive function of set shifting was practiced on *Two in One* (previously discussed), *Run Silent* 3, *Mission Decode,* and *Detective.* On *Run Silent* 3 the baseline score was 38 total errors. However, after practicing set shifting on *Two in One*, there was a significant generalization and the number of errors dropped to five. She approached zero errors by the sixth session, meeting the criterion of fewer than two errors on both trajectories (see Fig. 6.6). *Mission Decode* and *Detective* involved set shifting and reasoning/problem solving. Steady improvement was noted on *Mission Decode*, with one lapse on the seventh time she practiced the task. She met the criterion of not setting off the bomb twice in a row on trials eight and nine (see Fig. 6.7). On *Detective* 1 she learned to shift set and reason by analogy, such that she made no errors by Trial 6 (see Fig. 6.8). Figure 6.9 shows her performance on the more difficult Level 2 of *Detective*. She made steady progress, with one exception, until she committed no errors on the exercise. Reasoning was also practiced on *Spies*, on which she had to identify the figure that was "different" from the other three. Steady improvement can again be seen (Fig. 6.10).

Improved judgment based on attention to feedback was also practiced. Utilization of feedback was inherent in the set shifting exercises discussed above. Feedback on exercises that did not include set shifting was also undertaken. The exercises included *Number Guesser* 2, *Hid in the Grid*, and *Vocabulary.* On *Number Guesser* 2 (Fig. 6.11) she was eventually able to discover randomly generated four-digit numbers in only eight guesses based on feedback provided from her previous guesses. On *Hid in the Grid* she was initially unable to find the randomly located object within five guesses, but with practice she met this

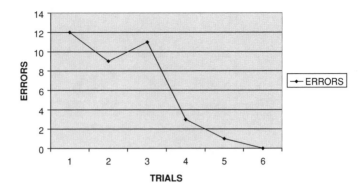

Fig. 6.8 AF executive functions: set shifting and reasoning on Detective 1

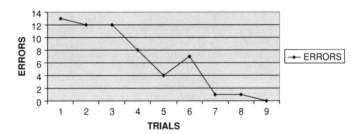

Fig. 6.9 AF executive functions: set shifting and reasoning on Detective 2

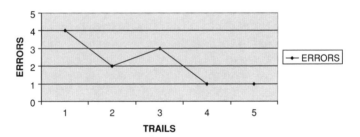

Fig. 6.10 AF executive functioning: visual–nonverbal reasoning on Spies

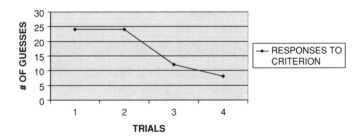

Fig. 6.11 AF executive functioning: effective use of feedback on Number Guesser 2

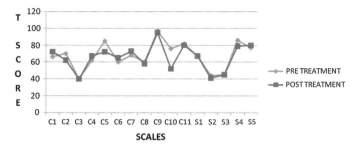

Fig. 6.12 AF LNNB performance

criterion four times in a row. On the easiest level of *Vocabulary* she required two or three clues per word and was able to correctly identify the words 50–87% of the time. This improved to 100% accuracy without requesting additional clues. On the intermediate level she required an average of two clues during the first practice session and had 80% accuracy. By the next session she scored 100% accuracy and required no clues beyond the initial ones provided. For each iteration of the exercise the computer randomly selected target words from a large pool of stimuli. Thus, skill generalization rather than memorization of specific stimuli accounted for improvement.

Application and integration of the elementary skills taught above were practiced on *Buying Power* and *What's My Name*. After memorizing the prices of goods and services on *Buying Power* 2, she was asked to determine the amount of change she should receive when paying specific amounts for particular goods and services she had memorized. She began with only 50% accuracy but soon moved to 100% accuracy. At baseline of *What's My Name* she was unable to learn all of the "peg word" prerequisites for the strategy taught, but after practice she learned and applied them such that she was able to remember 9 out of 10 names when confronted with the person's face.

After 17 months of treatment the patient was readministered the LNNB. Figure 6.12 graphically represents her pre- and post-test performance on LNNB. Probability levels were drawn from Table 14 in the LNNB manual. Attention on Clinical Scale 2 (C2) improved significantly from moderately impaired to mildly impaired ($p < 0.05$). Memory (C10) improved from moderately impaired to the normal range ($p < 0.01$). Improvement on the Intellectual Processes Scale (C11) did not reach statistical significance. No treatment was provided for arithmetic (C9) and motor functions (C1) and no statistically significant changes were seen following the intervention. This underscored the validity of treatment effects as described in the multiple baseline approach of Golden et al. The patient had been seeing a speech therapist but at the retesting her scores actually got worse (C5 and 6). This may be anomalous as her speech was much better prior to and following the post-treatment testing. Overall, brain impairment was slightly better (S4) and compensation (S5), was slightly worse but neither of these changes reached statistical significance.

She avoided perseverations on Controlled Oral Word Association (CFL) and an alternating figures task until she became fatigued, near the end of the tasks. Perseverations on Auditory Consonant Trigrams and Wisconsin Card Sorting were within normal limits. Divided attention on Trigrams was at the low end of normal for 9 and 36 seconds, and impaired at 18 seconds. On Wisconsin Card Sort she solved all six categories with a total of only 16 errors, reflecting excellent set shifting and problem solving.

Part way through treatment the patient began to walk her dog through the neighborhood so that she could meet and socially interact with her neighbors. At the conclusion of treatment the patient reapplied to the vocational rehabilitation program that had found her too impaired to qualify for their training. She was admitted, completed the program, and got a job placement on which she did well. She then moved from her mother's house into an assisted living program. She later returned to college and with allowances for extra time on exams received A's and B's in her coursework. She also returned to the last Day Treatment Center she had attended and volunteered to be an aide. The staff was amazed at her progress and pleased with her assistance and work with their current clients.

A second head trauma case was SB, a 24-year-old right-handed separated man with a high school education, who had an MVA. His car struck a barrel where there was roadwork and a boulder fell off the barrel and came through his windshield. He lost an eye and was comatose for some time. Initial workup revealed a Glasgow Coma Scale rating of 6. CT revealed skull fracture, pneumocephalus, subarachnoid hemorrhage, and multiple facial fractures. He underwent bifrontal craniotomy and oral facial surgery and spent 7 days in the ICU. The patient had anterograde and retrograde amnesia and lost 30 pounds. He was placed on Coumadin, Rebeprazide, and Depokote for mood swings.

About 1 month post injury he was transferred to a rehabilitation hospital for 3 weeks after which he was sent to another rehabilitation program. There he received Occupational Therapy for about a month after which he could perform activities of daily living. It was recommended he use a calculator and daily planner or Palm Pilot (i.e., prosthetic devices). He received Speech Therapy during the same period of time. At the end of 1 month he made many improvements but still had persisting problems in auditory comprehension, reading comprehension, and word finding. Attention and memory had not yet returned to normal levels.

Six months after his accident he was tested and found to have residual left hemisphere deficits, including naming disorder, problems generating words beginning with designated letters, vulnerability to interference when stimuli were verbal, verbal memory problems, inattention to verbal stimuli, and lower verbal IQ compared to performance IQ. One year after the accident he was again tested. Verbal learning and delayed verbal memory were still impaired but immediate verbal memory had returned to normal levels. Attention to verbal material was still impaired. He continued to demonstrate distractibility on verbal tasks (but not nonverbal ones). Visual naming improved to normal.

At this point a cognitive remediation program was devised to address his residual deficits. Baselines were taken 13 months after his injury. It was determined

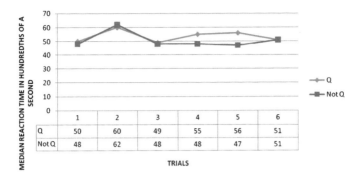

Fig. 6.13 SB alternating attention: Get Q 2

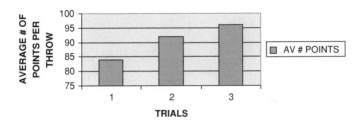

Fig. 6.14 SB focused and sustained attention: Space Probe 2 (1,400 points)

that attentional and executive problems could be practiced on several exercises upon which he performed below average. These were *Get Q* 2 (attention and set shifting in a verbal mode), *Two in One* 2, 3, and 4 (sustained attention, set shifting, mental operations, and impulse control with a verbal component), *Space Probe* (focused and sustained attention in a nonverbal mode), *Dartboard* 2 (sustained attention in a nonverbal mode), *Run Silent* 3 (set-shifting in a nonverbal mode), and *Double Trouble* (divided attention with verbal and nonverbal components). Focused attention on *Get Q* 1, set shifting on *Two in One* 1, and sustained attention and mental operations on *Type It* were within normal limits and not included in the treatment plan.

Figure 6.13 demonstrates that his response time on *Get Q* 2 was within normal limits except for the second trial. The number of errors never exceeded one, placing accuracy in the normal range. *Space Probe* exceeded the criterion of averaging more than 89 points per throw by the second trial when the goal was 1,400 points (see Fig. 6.14). The goal was increased to 9,999 points, but he had no difficulty maintaining the criterion performance (illustrated in Online Resource 1). Thus, sustained attention was demonstrated on this exercise.

Figure 6.15 reflects that speed on *Two in One* 2 was consistently within normal limits and on the last three trials, it was a full standard deviation above average. Accuracy was within or exceeded normal limits on the last three trials. Thus, speed and accuracy were average to above average on this task that required attention

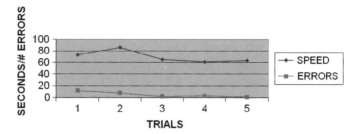

Fig. 6.15 SB sustained and alternating attention and impulse control: Two in One 2

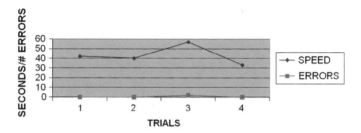

Fig. 6.16 SB sustained and alternating attention, mental manipulation and impulse control: Two in One ¾

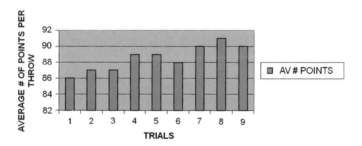

Fig. 6.17 SB sustained attention and visual motor tracking: Dartboard 2 (10,000 points)

and impulse control. When mental manipulation was added to this task, speed and accuracy remained normal over four trials (see Fig. 6.16).

Sustained attention on a fast moving visual-motor tracking task, *Dartboard* 2, met or exceeded the goal of averaging more than 89 points on the last three consecutive trials (see Fig. 6.17). The last five trials were undertaken 1 month after the first four trials because of a 1-month lapse in treatment due to his work-related travel. As can be seen in Fig. 6.17, his performance on trial 5 was equivalent to his performance on the last trial the month before (trial 4). On a similar task that added an alternating attention component, *Run Silent* 3, he achieved 100% accuracy on both trajectories by the seventh practice trial (see Fig. 6.18).

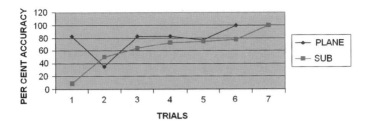

Fig. 6.18 SB alternating attention and visual motor tracking: Run Silent

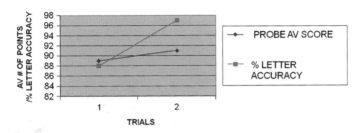

Fig. 6.19 SB sustained and divided attention: Double Trouble 1 (10,000 points)

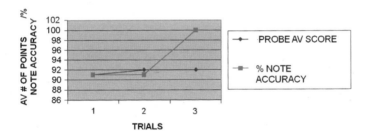

Fig. 6.20 SB sustained and divided attention: Double Trouble 2 (10,000 points)

The divided attention tasks were practiced to 10,000 points, adding a sustained attention element to the multitasking exercises. His *Double Trouble* 1 performance met the criterion in only two trials (see Fig. 6.19) while all scores met the criterion on *Double Trouble* 2, reflecting generalization of multitasking ability (see Fig. 6.20).

At this point his treatment was terminated and posttreatment testing was scheduled. Estimated intellectual functioning on LNNB improved from low average/average (IQ = 84–100) to average/above average (IQ = 94–110). Whereas he had previously perseverated on AVLT due to "forgetting" he had said the words, there was no perseveration following treatment. Other executive functions remained normal. Auditory focused attention was superior both before and after treatment. Visual attention on Stroop did not change, remaining average for nonverbal material and impaired for verbal material. Sustained visual attention

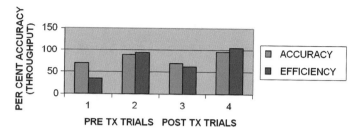

Fig. 6.21 SB sustained attention: pre and posttreatment ANAM performance

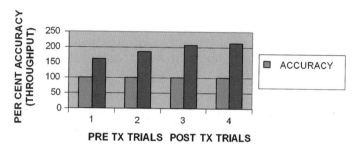

Fig. 6.22 SB focused visual attention: pre and posttreatment ANAM reaction time performance

Table 6.1 Pre and posttreatment delayed memory on AVLT in SB

Delayed recall	Delayed recognition
Pretreatment 6	Pretreatment 10
Posttreatment 10	Posttreatment 13

on the 1990s version of ANAM improved from the 12th percentile to the average range by the second posttreatment trial (see Fig. 6.21). Simple reaction time on the 1990s version of ANAM (focused visual attention) improved from below average (15–35th percentile) to average (41–44th percentile) for efficiency (see Fig. 6.22). Visual scanning and attention to numbers on Trails A improved from the 75th to the 86th percentile. Memory improved on AVLT in that he remembered what he said and no longer perseverated. Table 6.1 demonstrates that after a 30 minute delay AVLT recall improved from the 2nd percentile (impaired) to the 32nd percentile (average) and delayed recognition improved from below average (10–21st percentile) to average (54th percentile). Similarly, memory for designs on WMS III improved from the 25th percentile to the 61st percentile and recognition improved from the 75th percentile (average) to the 91st percentile (superior). Thus, attention training improved AVLT and Visual Reproduction performance. Strategies for story recall were not taught so, as expected, there was no change on Logical Memory. Likewise, motor awkwardness was not addressed and remained a problem on posttreatment testing. Again, the multiple baseline approach highlighted the efficacy of treatment in that targeted areas improved while non-targeted areas did not.

He was working full-time, enjoying his work, and was seen as a valuable contributor. His functioning was seen as comparable to the level displayed prior to the injury.

Another case of head trauma was WB, a 54-year-old woman who worked as an administrator in a position of authority in which she directed and supervised staff and her program. She was crossing the street when a speeding automobile hit her. She reportedly spun on top of the vehicle, her head hit and broke the car's windshield, and she was then thrown 30 feet into the street. She was not moving or breathing when the EMT arrived. She was unconscious for over 3 hours. Her first memory following the accident was finding herself in the emergency room of the hospital outside of which the accident had occurred. She had sustained a concussion and basilar skull fracture for which she was hospitalized for a 5 day observation. Symptoms included vertigo, loss of sense of smell, reduced sense of taste, short-term memory problems and "foggy" thinking.

Quantitative Electroencephalogram (QEEG) revealed slow (delta) activity in the left temporal area and excess delta, theta, and beta but minimal alpha waves. Visual evoked responses had only one significant asymmetry while auditory evoked responses had many significant deviations. The P300 wave revealed minimal problems but "could be better developed". The pattern of low amplitude electrical brain activity with eyes closed, increased slow activity and asymmetrical fast activity were compatible with postconcussion and cognitive problems. She was prescribed Ritalin and 2 months later Adderol was added to her regimen.

Neuropsychological testing was done 3 months postaccident. Results reflected residual problems in processing, perseveration, conceptual distractibility and flexibility, inferential reasoning, audioverbal encoding, and memory retrieval. It was recommended by her neuropsychologist that she be referred for cognitive remediation. She began this treatment 3 months after she had been tested, 6 months postinjury.

Her NeurXercise treatment plan addressed processing speed, attention, and perseveration on *Get Q*, *Two in One* and *Run Silent*. Memory was addressed on *Memory Game* Level 2, and *Symbol Memory*. Reasoning and set-shifting were approached through *Mission Decode*, *Detective*, and *Vocabulary*.

After 6 months of work on attention/processing speed and perseveration, she had improved enough to begin memory training in addition to continuing on attention. She met the criterion for normal performance in both attention and memory after two more months of training. She completed reasoning and set-shifting in 1 month.

Focused visual attention on *Get Q* 1 was practiced six times. Only one of the trials was outside of the normal range (see Fig. 6.23). Visual alternating attention is graphed in Online Resource 2. These results indicated that speed for accurate responding was improved to normal reaction time by the fifth session. The number of errors was erratic over the first four sessions but she made no errors during the fifth session (plotted on Online Resource 3). When the task was made more complex by adding more difficult discrimination among Q and non-Q stimuli (e.g., Q, O, G), she was able to keep her Q responses consistently within the range

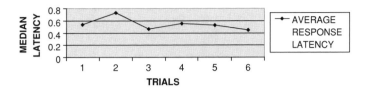

Fig. 6.23 WB focused visual attention: Get Q level 1

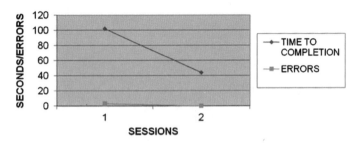

Fig. 6.24 WB sustained and alternating attention: Two in One level 1

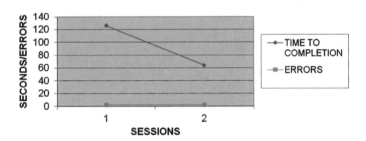

Fig. 6.25 WB sustained and alternating attention: Two in One level 2

of 0.60 seconds or less for Q (7 out of 8 sessions) and below 0.60 seconds for non-Qs (see Online Resource 4). She consistently made errors by responding to Qs as if they were similar looking letters. However, she did not respond to non-Qs as if they were Qs (see Online Resource 5). Her processing speed, attention, and freedom from perseveration were evident on the *Get Q* exercises.

After 2 months of working on the *Get Q* exercises, she returned to *Two in One*. Figures 6.24 and 6.25 show her baseline compared to her performance after working on *Get Q*. Generalization seemed to have taken place as she was well within normal limits following *Get Q* training but not before practicing those exercises. When a serial 3's alternating task was added to the *Two in One* paradigm (Levels 3 and 4), she had to work more but completed the task to criterion during the same session that she did on the other levels of *Two in One*. Figure 6.26 shows that baseline and her first practice trial were slow. Trial 1 represents her baseline score and the next 20 trials represent her work during a single session

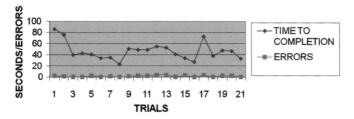

Fig. 6.26 WB sustained and alternating attention: Two in One ¾

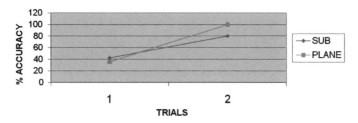

Fig. 6.27 WB alternating attention: Run Silent 3

about 2 months after baseline and following *Get Q* training. Trials 2–8 are her scores on *Two in One* Level 3 (all in normal range except for trial 2). The next eight trials represent the switch to Level 4. While she did not do as well as on Level 3 until she practiced for five trials, all scores were still within the normal range. She was then switched back to Level 3. She did poorly for the first trial of the switch and then returned to normal performance. She was switched to Level 4 again and she showed no deficit for three trials. Thus, processing speed, attention, and freedom from perseveration (set-shifting) were maintained.

Run Silent Level 3 was next practiced. The first trial in Fig. 6.27 represents her baseline and the next trial is her performance after two practice trials on Level 2 of *Run Silent*. She clearly maintained attention, processing speed, and freedom from perseveration (ability to alternate trajectories between targets).

She spent 6 months working on developing memory strategies to the point of scoring at the expected normal ranges on the exercises. Reasoning was within normal limits after working weekly on the exercises with the therapist over a 1-month period and at work daily during that time.

She was referred back to the neuropsychologist who had done the initial testing. He found significant improvement in visual attention to detail and consistency of visual–constructional reasoning. Visual processing was slightly more consistent and visual–constructional reasoning was more consistently above average than it had been prior to treatment. There was still some inefficiency on speeded tasks but there was a significant improvement from baseline. Divided attention showed a significant improvement, now being solidly average. Inferential reasoning in unstructured situations was improved. There was significant improvement in reasoning flexibility, with only the subtlest evidence of residual problems. Areas not targeted for treatment (e.g., auditory attention, tactile spatial recall, anosmia, and graphomotor speed) were unchanged from established pretreatment levels.

   She took charge of the amount of time she felt she could work based on her performance in treatment. She returned to work (10 hours per week) after she had been in treatment for 2 months. This was increased to 20 hours per week the next month and 30 hours per week 5 months thereafter. She returned to full-time employment the following month. She won back the respect and confidence of her staff and her superiors, although both groups had expressed some concern about her abilities when she first returned to work. She received superior job performance ratings and had the full confidence and support of her staff. She continued to work in her position for 4 years until her planned retirement. She and her husband had been building a home near their families in another State and they returned to that area and the new home upon her retirement.

Head Trauma Symptoms and Mechanisms

It should be clear that attention, memory, and executive functions are frequently impacted by head injury. All three were successfully addressed in the above cases and demonstrated generalization to the patients' lives at work, school, and in social settings. Mild head injuries usually involve concussion and diffuse axonal injury. More significant injuries, like those sustained by AF and SB, involve contusions and serious lesions of specific brain structures and regions. Damage is usually diffuse and bilateral in acceleration/deceleration injuries.

Blast Injuries

BI was a 58-year-old high ranking military officer injured in a blast when an improvised explosive device (IED) went off by the vehicle in which he was a passenger. Within a few hours of the blast he noticed neck and back pain, severe headache, dizziness, memory loss, confusion, pain in his teeth and shoulder, and problems with his bladder, sleep, and breathing. He was hospitalized and remained in ICU for 2 days after which he was confined to quarters on medication. Symptoms noted thereafter included marked dizziness, headaches, memory loss, slurred speech, attention deficit, cognitive fatigue, impaired concentration, name and word recall difficulties, and reading/writing problems. He was treated with vestibular rehabilitation for his dizziness, physical therapy, medication, craniosacral therapy, and acupuncture for the pain.

   He was tested 3 months after his injury and was found to be suffering from mild traumatic brain injury. His processing speed and motor speed were below expectations. Most areas of cognitive functioning were in the average range for this man whose premorbid functioning had been in the superior range. When he

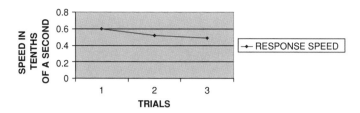

Fig. 6.28 BI focused attention/impulse control on Get Q level 1

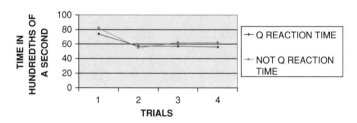

Fig. 6.29 BI alternating attention on Get Q 2

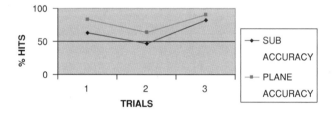

Fig. 6.30 BI alternating attention/set-shifting on Run Silent level 3

was offered no treatment for his cognitive problems, which did not demonstrate improvement over time, he began to research possible interventions. He got his physicians to make a referral for cognitive remediation 11 months after his blast injury. He added hyperbaric treatment to his regimen during the course of the cognitive remediation. Cognitive remediation treatment lasted 4 months and he had a follow-up appointment 4 months after the conclusion of cognitive remediation. He was still continuing his hyperbaric treatments at that time.

His treatment plan comprised the following. Focused attention/impulse control was practiced on *Get Q* 1, and alternating attention was practiced on *Get Q* 2 and *Run Silent* 3. Practice on visual attention required for *Run Silent* 3 was continued on *Dartboard* 2 to 1,000 points at speeds of 5 and 10. Facial memory was practiced on *Line Up* 2 and 3. Executive functions were practiced on *Mission Decode* 1 and 2 and *Double Trouble* 1 and 2.

His focused attention and impulse control improved from mildly impaired to the normal range in only three practice trials (see Fig. 6.28). Figures 6.29 and 6.30

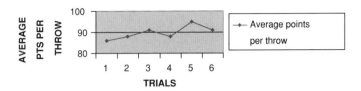

Fig. 6.31 BI visual attention and tracking on Dartboard level 2 (1,000 pts, speed = 5)

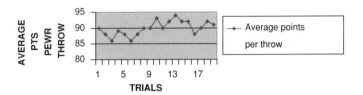

Fig. 6.32 BI visual attention and tracking on Dartboard 2 (1,000 pts, speed = 10)

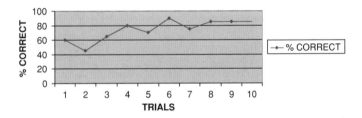

Fig. 6.33 BI facial memory on Line Up level 3

show that speed and consistency of alternating attention improved on *Get Q* 2 and *Run Silent* 3, respectively. He was able to consistently score above the criterion of 90 points per throw on another visual attention task, *Dartboard* 2, at two different tracking speeds (see Figs. 6.31 and 6.32).

Line Up 3 required identification of the target face from a line up of different faces, including a different photograph of the target from the one originally shown. In Fig. 6.33 it can be seen that his baseline was 60% correct. Between sessions 4 and 10 he dropped below 80% correct only twice. Matching to nonsample on *Line Up* 2 was harder for him. Baseline performance was 42% correct but he improved to 74% correct (see Fig. 6.34). Like Level 3, the targets changed randomly each time the exercise was practiced so there was no memorization effect. At the conclusion of treatment he was given the word list on *Memory Game* 2 for the first time. Having practiced and improved attention and facial memory, he scored 92% correct.

Executive functions were practiced on *Mission Decode* and *Double Trouble*. Online Resource 6 demonstrates a major improvement in executive function from baseline to the first trial on *Mission Decode* 1. He was able to meet the criterion of not exploding before completing the series of problems on the last three trials of

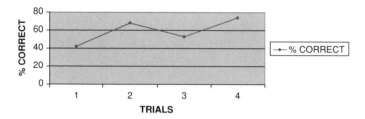

Fig. 6.34 BI facial memory on Line Up level 2

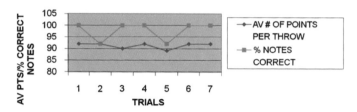

Fig. 6.35 BI multitasking on Double Trouble level 2 (1,600 pts)

Mission Decode 2 (see Online Resource 7). Another exercise that involved executive functioning was *Double Trouble*, which practiced divided attention/multitasking. On Level 1 he practiced to 600 points per trial and was able to throw the optimal number of darts on trials 2–4 and simultaneously respond to the letters with one or no misses on the last two trials (see Online Resource 8). He had difficulty with multitasking on *Double Trouble* 2 and aborted his first five attempts at the exercise. Online Resource 9 tracks his completed trials and does not include his initial or additional aborted trials. Practicing to 600 points, he was consistent in averaging over 80 points per throw and correctly responding to the tones at the same time. The criterion was then increased to 1,600 points, requiring him to practice more than twice as long per trial. Figure 6.35 reflects that performance was consistently excellent, exceeding 90 points per throw on six of seven trials and generally at 100% correct notes. The criterion was then raised to 3,000 points per trial and he scored 91 points per throw on average and 100% correct response to notes. Thus, his multitasking became more accurate for a period that was five times as long as the initial period required for him to perform.

Posttreatment testing revealed that attention improved on Letter Number Sequencing from average to superior while Digit Symbol, Trails A, and Conners' CPT remained average. Memory was superior on Logical Memory I and II. CVLT II under cuing conditions demonstrated an improvement from 2 to 4 words more that were retrieved spontaneously. Recognition on CVLT II improved from 13 out of 16 words to 16 out of 16 words. Immediate and delayed recall on CVLT II did not change from the average range. Executive functioning improved overall. Abstract reasoning on Similarities improved from average to superior. Multi-tasking on Auditory Consonant Trigrams was average, above average, and average on the three trials before treatment but improved to superior, superior, and above average, respectively, following treatment. Proactive Interference on CVLT II improved from average to above average but retroactive interference remained below average. Testing results suggested that there was some gain in all areas targeted for treatment but several measures did not show improvement.

In terms of ecological validity, he and his wife reported that his memory was much improved on a day-to-day basis. He could again express his thoughts articulately most of the time. His processing speed was noted to have improved, according to his wife and himself (this is consistent with PASAT score being above average on the fastest, most demanding trial). A few months after treatment terminated he was again able to handle high level briefs for hours at a time. However, he then became depleted and suffered dizziness, confusion, fatigue, and headaches. The depletion effect lasted 1–3 days. He experienced one such episode during the treatment phase and at least two others after completing cognitive remediation. A few months after the last episode he attended a week-long conference and participated actively with little fatigue throughout the week. He had returned to work on a part-time basis and thereafter resumed his profession full-time. Thus, he made excellent improvement and this continued over time following formal treatment sessions.

ZW was a 23-year-old enlisted serviceman with a high school education and reported grade point average of 2.5. He reported he was exposed to 50 IED blasts over three deployments. He had three episodes of loss of consciousness. He was screened about a year after his last loss of consciousness, and tested 1 month later and then 4 months after that. He remained in cognitive remediation treatment for 5 months and stopped when his attention scores were consistently in the normal range on NeurXercise. He dropped out of psychotherapy while he was still symptomatic for sequelae of posttraumatic stress disorder (PTSD).

Initial complaints included headaches, extreme fatigue, attention problems, short-term memory loss, and insomnia. He reported blurred vision, tinnitus, sensorimotor problems, language difficulty, and planning/organizing problems. Pretreatment testing revealed intellectual functioning to be below average, immediate and delayed list memory to be impaired, and list learning was likewise impaired. Immediate and delayed story memory was intact. Visual attention was impaired while auditory attention was excellent. Executive functions, sensorimotor skills, constructional ability, academic skills, and language were all intact.

Visual attention was targeted using *Get Q, Two in One, Dartboard*, and *Run Silent*. Multitasking was targeted using *Double Trouble*. Memory was not targeted pending the evaluation of change due to improved attention.

Focused and sustained visual attention and impulse control were practiced on *Get Q* Level 1 and *Dartboard*. Visual alternating attention was practiced on *Get Q* 2 and *Run Silent*. Divided attention was practiced on *Double Trouble*. The baseline of *Get Q* 1 was marred by impulsivity (errors at speeds too fast to have been visually processed). His baseline was about 0.83 seconds whereas his target was set for below 0.60 seconds without impulsive responding. After about a month of practice he was averaging 0.65 seconds. He was highly variable thereafter, with median scores as good as 0.58 seconds and as slow as 0.72 seconds. He finally completed the exercise averaging less than 0.50 seconds as his median response speed. Baselines on *Get Q* 2 for visual alternating attention were slow overall but also inaccurate due to occasional impulsive responding. By the second treatment session (having practiced *Get Q* 1 for months), he was responding to non-Qs within the target range but was still a little slow on Qs (median response time was 0.66 seconds). The following session he was able to respond to Qs and non-Qs faster than a median of 0.60 seconds for three consecutive iterations of the exercise, each lasting about 5 minutes. Two weeks later he demonstrated excellent performance when *Get Q* 1 was reintroduced to ensure that he had not lost ground (he averaged less than 0.50 seconds per response). The following week he demonstrated continuing improvement on *Get Q* 2 (about 0.45 seconds for Qs and non-Qs for the last two practice iterations of that session).

The following week he began *Two in One* Level 1. Three of four practice trials were faster than the mean for unimpaired individuals and the remaining trial was within a standard deviation of the mean (baseline was more than a standard deviation below the mean). Only one of three practice trials on Level 2 was outside of the average range (his baseline was over three standard deviations below average). Four more trials at Level 1 produced above average scores with no errors on three of the trials and one error on the other. Level 3 was also practiced during the same session and while baseline was more than a standard deviation below average, he was close to the median on one trial and almost two standard deviations above the mean on the second trial. The work on *Get Q* seemed to have generalized to his performance on this second visual alternating attention task.

He scored in the normal range on *Run Silent* 1 and 2 and proceeded to Level 3 on which baseline scores from 4 months earlier were 31 and 65% accuracy for the two trajectories. This jumped to 83 and 70%, followed by 82 and 91%, and finally 83 and 82%. The last two trials met the criterion of no more than two misses on each trajectory. The following week he averaged over 90 points per throw on *Dartboard* 1 and 2, meeting the criterion on that exercise. He next undertook divided attention with *Double Trouble*. At baseline he scored 60 points per throw and 60% correct letters on Level 1 and 56 points per throw with 57% correct notes on Level 2. Having practiced the other attention exercises to criterion, he scored 85 points per throw and 100% correct letters at a faster than baseline pace on Level 1. He was then administered the exercise at that faster, more demanding speed for almost twice as long. He scored 84 points with 80% correct letters.

Following cognitive remediation of his attention problems he was retested. He no longer reported fatigue, handwriting problems, or difficulty climbing stairs. He continued to complain of the other problems he had described above. Some of these appeared to be related to his emotional difficulties, the treatment for which he had not completed.

Estimated level of intelligence on the Luria-Nebraska was below average pre and posttreatment. The LNNB has two measures of effort and both indicated he was making a reasonable effort on this neuropsychological battery. He received no cognitive remediation on the areas tested by the intellectual scale of the LNNB.

Memory on AVLT was worse on the first presentation but over the five trials he improved from the 2nd percentile in the pretreatment phase to the 13th percentile at posttreatment testing. Immediate memory for the Luria story was within normal limits both pre and posttreatment. Delayed memory on AVLT improved from the 2nd percentile to the 19th percentile and was borderline normal on the LNNB pre and posttreatment. Story recall after 15 minutes was borderline normal both times and memory for a design improved from three of 10 parts recalled in pretreatment after a delay to five parts of ten recalled. Memory, which had not been directly targeted, was still outside of normal limits but his score on all three trials of the TOMM raised questions about his motivation to do well on visual memory tasks. Visual attention, which was targeted and on which he performed well within normal limits over the training, showed no improvement on retesting. Stroop and Trails A remained Impaired while auditory attention measures remained unchanged (PA-SAT was still superior and LNNB was still above average). Language scores remained within normal limits but visual perception and spatial skills got worse although no new event had intervened. While secondary gain could not be ruled out as an explanation for the decrement in his visual and spatial performance, emotional issues could also account for his ineffective and inconsistent performance.

He was placed on temporary medical retirement. He did not make any further contact and it could not be determined how he fared after he left treatment.

GA was a 21-year-old high school graduate enlisted military serviceman who sustained a blast injury with right parietal intracranial hemorrhage. He denied loss of consciousness. He was hospitalized, found to have attention, memory and visual spatial problems on screening, and was given a full neuropsychological testing battery 3 months later. Complaints at the time of the full testing included hearing problems and memory difficulties. He denied sensorimotor, visual, attention, language, and executive problems.

On the LNNB only spelling and reading were outside of the normal range. Focused auditory attention on LNNB was above average and sustained auditory attention on PASAT was average, consistent with the results of the P300 auditory evoked potential test administered by the Neurology department. However, visual attention was far below average on Stroop (1–6th percentiles) and Trails A (8th percentile). While immediate memory was within normal limits on LNNB, it was at the 7th percentile on AVLT. Executive functioning was variable. Multitasking on Auditory Consonant Trigrams was variable (9th, 45th, and 10th percentiles). Freedom from interference was average on AVLT (34–37th percentiles) and Stroop (50th percentile). Set-shifting on Trails B was far below expectancy (8th percentile). Freedom from perseveration on PASAT was excellent. He was concrete when giving definitions, explaining proverbs, or responding to how things were similar or different. He began cognitive remediation 6 months thereafter (9 months post injury).

Visual alternating attention was targeted with *Get Q* 2, *Two in One*, and *Run Silent*. Executive functions were targeted with *Double Trouble* (multitasking).

On *Get Q* 2 responses to non-Qs were accurate and within normal limits but variable and with errors on Qs during the baseline. Over the course of the first session, performance did not improve. He was unable to return for a month before resuming treatment. Performance was usually within normal processing speed for Q and non-Qs but always with errors during the first session upon his return. By the end of the following session he had responded to Qs and non-Qs within expected speeds and without errors for two consecutive iterations of the exercise. He was then out for another month before returning to treatment. His baseline was within normal limits on *Two in One* 1 but slow and marked with errors on Levels 2 and 3. When he returned to treatment (2 months after the baseline had been collected), he began with slight improvement in time and accuracy over baseline but after seven trials had succeeded in demonstrating normal performance for accuracy and speed on two consecutive trials. During that same session he began to work on Level 3. He was accurate and demonstrated normal speed on the first two efforts he made on this level and was felt to have succeeded, with apparent generalization from the previous level he had practiced. Baseline performance on *Run Silent* 3 was 62.5 and 40% accuracy on the two trajectories, respectively. On his very first attempt following success on *Get Q* and *Two in One*, his performance improved to 72.7 and 90.9%. The following session began with his having only one miss on each of the trajectories, thus meeting the criterion that had been set for success.

Double Trouble was next presented to work on the executive skill of multitasking. Speed of presentation was kept the same as the baseline speed but the exercise was set to last almost twice as long as it had during baseline collection. After 3 weeks Level 1 was consistently performed within normal limits (averaging over 90 points per launch and not more than one error). After 2 weeks he was able to consistently average over 90 points per launch and respond accurately to the notes on Level 2. Thus, he had met the criteria for success on all exercises set for his treatment plan and he was retested.

Spelling improved a full standard deviation back into the normal range on LNNB, suggesting that attention rather than spelling problems were the etiology of his poor pretreatment performance in this area. Reading remained impaired and unchanged. While auditory attention on PASAT had been average on pretreatment testing (48th percentile), it improved to the 73rd percentile, suggesting he was much more efficient following treatment. Visual processing speed tested out worse on Trails A (10 seconds slower) and Stroop (from 1–12th percentiles to 1–8th percentiles). However, Trails B, which requires visual processing speed complicated by alternating attention, showed improvement from 8th to 39th percentile. Immediate memory on AVLT improved from 7th percentile to 21st percentile, suggesting that attention had been part of the problem but not completely the cause of his immediate memory difficulty. On executive functioning, multitasking was targeted for treatment. Performance on Trigrams improved from 9–45th percentiles to 31–44th percentiles. Set shifting improved on Trails B from the 8th to the 39th percentile. Freedom from interference had not been targeted and did not improve. To evaluate the extent to which PTSD might be interfering with his cognitive functioning, he was administered the PAI and DAPS. Both strongly indicated he was still suffering the effects of PTSD even though he and his psychotherapist felt he had made improvement in this area.

His cognitive improvement and reduction in PTSD symptoms allowed him to return to full duty. It was recommended he continue his psychotherapy to reduce further the symptoms of PTSD and dysthymia.

SP was a 22 year-old enlisted military member who had exposure to three IED blasts during his 3 year military service, with no reported symptoms. Then he suffered a penetrating head injury from mortar blast, leaving schrapnel embedded in his head. He was comatose for a month. During that time he underwent a craniotomy but this failed to remove all of the shrapnel fragments embedded in his frontal lobes and brainstem. He also developed an aneurysm, necessitating further surgery and stent of the left middle cerebral artery. He was sent home for 2 weeks during which time he was seen at a local VA hospital for neuropsychological testing. He was found to have deficits in "focused simple attention, verbal fluency when prompted with a phonemic cue and recall of visual information".

He then returned to the military hospital for 2 months before transferring for 1 month to an inpatient rehabilitation facility. At the rehabilitation program he was taught relaxation techniques to help with pain management and to write down things he needed to remember as a compensation for his memory problems (i.e., use of a prosthetic device rather than developing compensation through alternate functional systems). He then returned to the military hospital for an additional month. He underwent numerous surgeries to remove as much of the schrapnel from his brain as could be done without endangering his life. In addition to a neurosurgeon, he was followed by a neurologist and psychiatrist who were treating his pain and emotional symptoms. About 2 months later he was retested by a neuropsychologist. Symptoms at that time included head pain, dizziness, post-traumatic stress symptoms, anxiety, insomnia, deficits in attention/concentration, memory problems, comprehension difficulties, and becoming easily confused. He was medicated with Topomax, Seroquel and Paxil. Test findings reflected significant inattention, verbal fluency problems, and executive dysfunction. Immediate and delayed memory problems were believed to be significantly impacted by the attention deficit. He was referred for cognitive remediation at that time (about 8 months post injury) to address the attention, memory, and executive problems.

Inattention was addressed with *Two in One*, *Get Q*, *Dartboard*, and *Run Silent*. Memory problems were targeted with *Line Up*, *Memory Game*, and *Symbol Memory*. Executive functions were to be practiced on *Foreign Intrigue*, *Strategy*, and *Double Trouble*. However, he moved across country before the executive functions could be addressed.

He practiced *Get Q* Level 1 but this was discontinued after two sessions as he became frustrated having to wait for the target to appear on an infrequent basis. After 2 months of practicing *Get Q* Level 2 he had improved his reaction time from over one second to each stimulus to about 0.8 seconds for each. He then continued to practice this exercise as well as others so that he would not be too bored from doing the same exercise exclusively. Three months thereafter he was still variable, but at times averaged better than 0.7 seconds for both Q and not Q.

On *Two in One* Level 1 he was able to reach the normal range in the first two sessions after baseline and moved on to Level 2. Within a single session he improved to the normal range on Level 2. After five sessions he performed in the normal range on the more difficult Levels 3 and 4, which include the executive function of mental operations as well as focused and alternating attention. He reached criterion on *Dartboard* in two of six trials within a single session. The following session he scored over 90 points on average for the first two practice trials so the target was deemed met. He then began to work on *Run Silent* Level 3. After two practice sessions he was still performing with much difficulty so training began on Level 1, practicing only firing at the plane. He was accurate on only 50% of his firings on the first trial but had only one miss in the next trial. He then practiced Level 2, only dropping bombs. In three practice trials he was performing accurately (2 misses out of 12 bombs dropped). He then returned to practice firing on the plane again to ensure he could continue to do this accurately. In fact, he had regressed and did not perform well initially. As he did better, he was switched to the other trajectory and had problems again. After about 3 weeks he was able to perform well with each trajectory by itself. He was then moved to Level 3 again.

After practicing *Run Silent* for a while he was able to improve his score on *Dartboard* from a baseline average of 76 points per throw to 90 points per throw (the target that had been set for him). He eventually could perform *Run* Silent with only three misses on each trajectory. He then attempted to perform the same task using a more complex and difficult approach that involved hitting the sub and plane during the same pass instead of doing each consecutively. He was able to succeed with five or six misses on this task that he had devised although I had not thought it possible to perform the exercise this way.

He then began to work on memory with *Memory Game* Level 2. His baseline was 36% recall of the words containing strings of three and four words. He eventually improved to 75% correct for strings of five, six, and seven words, using the strategies he was taught. The speed was slowed considerably so that he could practice the strategies multiple times and then immediately retrieve the words. He reached 100% retention. Once he could do this consistently, the exposure/practice time was gradually reduced while working on his retaining the words.

Nonverbal memory was practiced on *Symbol Memory*. He was able to consistently recall and recognize 5 out of 6 symbols by using the strategies he was taught and occasionally he could recall all six symbols. Facial memory on *Line Up* Level 1 improved from 13 of 19 faces recalled to 18 of 19.

He had been tested prior to his leaving the area and 1 year after that. His posttreatment scores on measures of attention were unchanged and still reflected poor performance. Conners' CPT showed the same 4 of 7 inattention measures to be abnormal. Visual tracking and processing speed on Trails A improved 0.7 standard deviations but was still significantly impaired. Visual and nonverbal attention and processing speed on Stroop remained below the 1st percentile. RBANS remained impaired on the Attention subtest on both Forms A and B. Impulsivity/perseveration on CPT reflected impulsivity on one of three measures when pretreatment scores reflected no impulsivity. Card Sort perseveration scores improved from below average (16th percentile) to the average range (58th percentile). Trails B was below the 1st percentile on both testings. One year later attention on these measures was relatively unchanged. Trails A had improved from below the 1st percentile to the 5th percentile. CPT reflected problems on five inattention measures compared to four before and after treatment. Stroop remained impaired as did the RBANS attention subtest. Impulsivity on Conners' demonstrated diminished functioning, from no impulsivity before treatment to 1 of 3 measures positive for impulsivity to all three measures positive for impulsivity. Trails B improved from below the 1st percentile to the 1st percentile, not suggesting much of an improvement. His ability to maintain his attention continued to be affected by the interaction of PTSD, depression, and brain damage.

Immediate memory functioning on RBANS was impaired (below the 1st percentile) before and after treatment but improved to Borderline (5th percentile) 1 year post cognitive remediation. Delayed memory on RBANS, however, was below the 1st percentile for all three evaluations. Delayed list memory on RBANS was 0 of 10 recalled after treatment and 2 of 10 recalled 1 year later (on an alternate form of RBANS). However, recognition memory after the delay was 8 of 20 after treatment and 17 of 20 a year later (using form A the year before and form B on the 1 year follow-up). Thus, recognition memory had improved significantly and the result suggested that encoding and consolidation were much better while retrieval remained a problem. Story recall after the delay was essentially the same (6 of 12 facts recalled versus 5 a year earlier). He forgot most of the complex figure on RBANS the year before (earning 1 point out of 20), whereas he did somewhat better in 1 year follow-up (5 points out of 20).

Intellectual functioning on WASI improved from Borderline to below average following treatment and stayed at the below average level 1 year later. However, performance was highly inconsistent and erratic, suggesting attentional problems disrupted performance on different subtests on different occasions. For example, Similarities scores varied from 7th percentile to 33rd percentile and back down to 16th percentile. Matrix Reasoning went from average to borderline and back to average.

Language was not treated during his cognitive remediation and his RBANS Language subtest scores remained at the borderline level. His language was addressed by speech therapy in the intervening year, but they did not see much in the way of progress and his testing scores remained in the borderline range. Constructional skills were untreated and remained in the impaired range on RBANS throughout the three testings (Forms A, B, and A, respectively).

During the course of treatment his sense of humor returned, he became more trusting, began to date a woman he fell in love with, and married and they decided to buy a home out of state. He became less stubborn, more cognitively flexible and hence more cooperative with treatment recommendations. His memory and executive functioning improved to the point that he usually called if he could not keep an appointment, in sharp contrast to the first several months of treatment when he frequently missed without notification and could not remember where he put the appointment reminder notices that he had. For almost the entire first year of treatment he could not complete a session without experiencing a debilitating headache. By the conclusion of treatment he was usually able to complete the session without headaches disrupting his performance or causing a premature end to the session.

When he moved out of state, he entered an outpatient rehabilitation program and his PTSD and head pain were targeted. During the intervening year he contacted his cognitive remediation therapist on several occasions and asked for his therapist to consult with the rehabilitation program around areas he felt were not showing progress. The program was very open to input and eager to find new ways to try to help SP. When he returned for retesting a year later, his PTSD symptoms had still failed to remit but he had just recently been put on a sustained release pain medication that was helping his pain level. He spoke about the possibility of getting biofeedback for his head pain when he returned to his home.

Blast Injury Symptoms and Mechanisms

The mechanisms involved in blast injury to the brain are thought to be quite different from the acceleration/deceleration mechanism discussed in the head trauma section. Some hypotheses include overpressure and shock waves. Neurological and cognitive effects of blast injuries have not yet been characterized in the research literature. However, the following represents my clinical experience with this population. In the acute phase most patients exposed to blasts "appear" to have no cognitive deficits and interact relatively normally with their doctors. However, formal neuropsychological testing reveals that a portion of them perform abnormally, especially in the areas of visual–spatial functioning and word generation. Some also show deficits in memory, attention, and executive functioning. These observations are similar to those in the composite examples of blast injured individuals reported by French et al. (2010). Many show significant improvement over the next few months but some do not fully recover without intervention. The cases reviewed herein suggested that the mildly impaired patients with postacute residual cognitive problems responded well to cognitive remediation and were able to make significant improvement in their daily lives. Problems that persisted into the postacute phase were visual but not auditory attention, processing speed, and executive functions, including multitasking. SP was by all definitions severely impaired, with 1 month loss of consciousness and significant retrograde amnesia. He also had a complicated picture that included embedded schrapnel and multiple neurosurgeries in addition to blast exposure, PTSD, and pain. Nonetheless, he made great strides in his ability to interact, develop a relationship and follow through with treatment recommendations. These real-life changes were in contrast to his failure to show meaningful improvements on the neuropsychological measures and raised questions about the interfering role of PTSD and pain when neurological functioning had perhaps shown some improvement. All of the above cases had factors that complicated the picture of blast injury, including physical and psychological problems, possible secondary gain, and more than one type of neurological mechanism of injury (e.g., blast plus PTSD and pain, HUMVEE rollover, or blunt head injury). Therefore, it is more difficult to separate the blast effects from the effects of the concomitant problems. A similar conclusion was drawn by MacDonald et al. (2011) who found multiple mechanisms of injury in the blast-exposed soldiers they evaluated.

Stroke

Patients who suffered strokes as part of a more complicated neurological picture are discussed in other sections of this book (e.g., RB under Subcortical Disorders, KP under Co-morbid Conditions). Patient CVA suffered a stroke without other complications and will be discussed in this section.

CVA was a 57-year-old man who suffered a stroke about 7 months before he was due to retire from a high level position in the military. The cerebrovascular accident was in the posterior fossa and was caused by an arteriovenous malformation (AVM). The stroke left him severely ataxic and with dysarthria. He awoke one day with right-sided facial and body weakness. CT revealed posterior fossa hemorrhage. An angiogram revealed left-sided AVM. The AVM was embolized and he was noted to have severe ataxia, dysarthria, and dysphagia. He received intensive inpatient physical, occupational, and speech therapy. MRI of the brain taken about 1 month post-stroke revealed parenchymal hemorrhage in the vermis and bilateral cerebellar hemispheres, infarct in right inferior occipital and superior cerebellar hemispheres, and small separate right frontal deep white matter infarct. Echocardiogram at that time was normal. He was able to ambulate with a walker and use a cane. Speech was still marked with paraphasias and the need for leading questions to get him to communicate effectively.

Multiple MRIs were done over the next several years. Four years following the stroke his MRI revealed encephalomalacia involving right greater than left cerebellum vermis and inferior right temporal lobe. There were also scattered punctate lacunar lesions. He received neuropsychological testing three times over the first 4 years since the stroke. Four years after the stroke he had deficits in confrontational naming, lexical and semantic fluency, right manual motor ability, spatial organization, sustained attention, and executive functions. Five months after this last testing (i.e., 4.5 years post stroke) he began cognitive remediation to address attention, spatial organization, right hand manual motor skill, and executive problems.

Attention training included *Two in One* Levels 1, 2, 3, and 4, *Get Q* Level 2, and *Run Silent* Level 3. Motor rehabilitation was addressed by use of the right hand on *Get Q* 2, *Two in One* and *Double Trouble*. Spatial organization was addressed on *Run Silent* and *Double Trouble*. Executive functions were practiced on *Double Trouble*, *Detective* Levels 1 and 2, and *Mission Decode* Levels 1 and 2.

He was able to improve his speed on *Two in One* Level 1 from four standard deviations below average to the average range (Fig. 6.36). His baseline was 176 seconds and nine errors (not shown on graph). The figure shows his improvement over three practice sessions on consecutive weeks beginning 2 weeks after the baseline was taken. He used his unimpaired left hand to perform the task. Figure 6.37

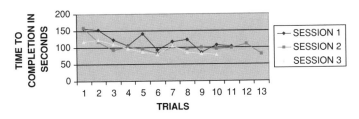

Fig. 6.36 CVA alternating attention on Two in One level 1

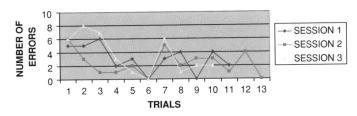

Fig. 6.37 CVA accuracy of alternating attention on Two in One level 1

reflects the accuracy of the above performance on the three sessions. Errors were within normal limits on approximately one third of the trials on the first session and approximately half of the second and third sessions. He was then instructed to practice using both hands as his homework assignment (motor skill rehabilitation), with the plan being to eventually achieve scores comparable to Figs. 6.36 and 6.37.

After practicing with both hands during the week and during the next session, he was able to bring his scores into the range he had reached using his left hand only. Advancing to Level 2 during that same session and using both hands he was able to get one trial within normal speed out of 12 attempts. Only 5 of the 12 trials were two standard deviations below normal speed. He practiced this exercise over the next week. After an additional 2 weeks he scored within a standard deviation of normal and most errors were motor control related rather than cognitive.

He then began Get Q Level 2. He was slow responding to Qs (median response time of 0.85 seconds) but within normal limits responding to not-Qs (0.56 seconds). He returned 2 weeks later and scored a median of 0.65 for Q and 0.61 for not-Q (consistent on both targets, reflecting good alternating attention).

At this point he was begun on *Run Silent*. Accuracy was 33–50%. He was gone for about a month before resuming, although he practiced on his laptop while he was away. On his return he began the session with 66–83% accuracy and ended the session with 9 hits out of 11 tries on the planes and 10 hits out of 11 tries on the subs (82–91% accuracy). He then returned to *Two in One* Level 2 in this same session and was able to score close to the mean for unimpaired individuals after five practice sessions. All of the five practice sessions had been about one standard deviation from the mean as had been his previous performance on this exercise, but his improvement to near the mean thereafter reflected a significant improvement in attention. He completed the session practicing *Two in One* Level 3.

When he returned the next week the answers to Level 3 had become automated so he was switched to Level 4, a comparable serial 3's task starting with 2B instead of 1A. As expected, his score returned to the baseline demonstrated in the last session before he memorized the sequence. He flipped back and forth during that session until he could perform each level at the speed and accuracy of unimpaired individuals without resorting to automatization. The interference effect of switching between the two levels prevented automatization and this was noted in his calculating aloud instead of quickly typing the responses. At this point the attention training was deemed complete.

He next worked on executive functioning with *Double Trouble*. After two sessions he was able to consistently average over 90 points per launch while responding correctly to either all letters or all tone pairs while firing his rockets. He returned in 2 weeks and completed *Mission Decode* on Level 1 and began Level 2. The following week he got 20 of 40 correct on Level 2 and the week after that was able to pass Level 2 with 36 out of 40 correct answers. During that same session he passed *Detective* Level 1 with 17 out of 20 correct answers.

He returned for repeat neuropsychological testing with the following results. Visual attention improved on Trails A from about the 34th percentile ($T = 46$) to the upper end of the average range (72nd percentile). Digit Symbol-Coding was unchanged. Auditory attention was essentially unchanged on Digit Span and Letter Number Sequencing, remaining within normal limits. Spatial skills were re-evaluated on Block Design (no change from average) and Rey Complex Figure copy, which was Impaired at pretreatment (2nd percentile) but within normal limits (35/36 segments correct) at posttreatment. Visual Reproduction copy was superior (95th percentile). Repeat testing on Grooved Pegboard revealed his right hand performance improved from severely impaired below the 1st percentile ($T = 17$) to below average (22nd percentile). Executive functioning was improved on Trails B, from about the 18–19th percentile ($T = 41$) to 54th percentile. Abstract reasoning on Similarities improved from SS $= 8$ (25th percentile) to SS $= 10$ (50th percentile). Memory and language were not treated with NeurXercise and there were no changes from average on Immediate and Delayed Logical Memory and Immediate Visual Reproduction. However, delayed Visual Reproduction improved from above average to superior. For language, Boston Naming remained Borderline/mildly impaired, Animal Fluency improved from the 9th percentile to the 18th percentile and there was little change on FAS ($T = 36$; 8th percentile versus 11th percentile). Thus, it appears that the changes in areas targeted were valid indicators of the effectiveness of the specific treatments as there was little change in the areas not targeted by the treatment.

Ecological validity was demonstrated by his spontaneously using the right hand most of the time, his reports of finding his way around more easily (spatial organization) and improved ability to pay attention. His wife, an occupational therapist, felt he had made dramatic improvements since undertaking cognitive remediation. He requested permission to make a copy of the program disk as he found the exercises enjoyable and challenging and wished to continue to work with them on his own.

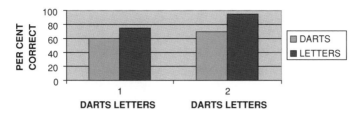

Fig. 6.38 RF divided attention-Double Trouble level 1

Stroke Symptoms and Mechanisms

Residual symptoms are likely to be present and need remediation if recovery has not taken place over the first 3–6 months post stroke. Symptoms will vary, depending on the region affected by the cardiovascular accident. For example, CVA had infarcts in the cerebellar, temporal, and occipital regions, leading to symptoms affecting balance, motor control, and spatial organization. Attention and executive problems suggested that there was also likely some frontal lobe compromise.

Neurosurgical Intervention

RF was a 45-year-old college educated computer programmer. He had neurosurgical removal of a right frontal meningioma 8 years prior to cognitive remediation and had been suffering from memory, attention, and information processing problems since the surgical intervention. A year and a half prior to his seeking cognitive remediation, he was diagnosed with a left frontal meningioma, but it was not recommended that he have surgery.

Eight years postsurgery neuropsychological testing revealed below average or impaired performance in visual motor skills, attention/scanning, auditory vigilance, information processing speed, divided attention, word generation, and new verbal learning. Further, many of his "average" scores were also felt to be below his premorbid functioning and therefore reflective of cognitive inefficiency.

His treatment program was aimed at improving attention, processing speed, spatial skills, memory, and reasoning. Attention and processing speed were practiced until he reached normal performance levels on *Get Q* 1 and 2, and *Two in One* 1–4. *Double Trouble* is a divided attention task that requires attention, processing speed, and spatial skill. He was able to improve spatial skills by 10% while simultaneously attending to and improving on *Get Q* to 95% accuracy from 75% accuracy at pretreatment baseline (Fig. 6.38).

Memory and list learning were treated with *Memory Game 2*. Facial memory training employed *Line Up* 3 and *What's My Name*. Online Resource 10 reflects that he learned a total of 75 words after being taught strategies compared to 50 words at pretreatment baseline. On *Line Up* 3 the target faces changed randomly

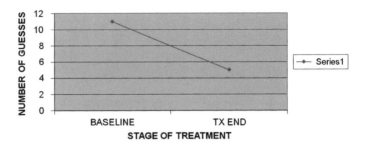

Fig. 6.39 RF reasoning-Number Guesser level-2

every time the exercise was practiced so that memorizing the correct answer did not become an issue. Online Resource 11 shows that at pretreatment baseline he recognized 60% of the targets when presented with different poses from the target pose. Following treatment he was 98% accurate. Remembering name–face pairings on *What's My Name* improved from 40% at pretreatment to 90% following practice using the peg-word system (Online Resource 12).

Reasoning was approached through *Vocabulary, Number Guesser* 2, *Mission Decode* and *Detective*. Online Resource 13 demonstrates that guessing words based on clues improved from 40% at baseline to 100% following training. Generating guesses and utilizing feedback to improve performance and derive correct solutions on *Number Guesser* 2 showed significant improvement with treatment (Fig. 6.39), from an average of 11 guesses to an average of five guesses. Target numbers were always different for every presentation. Therefore, improvement could only occur by learning a reasoning process and not by memorizing previous answers. Performance on *Mission Decode* (Online Resource 14) improved from 10% correct to 100% correct answers. *Detective* (Online Resource 15) improved from 60 to 100% accuracy.

Table 6.2 summarizes pretreatment and posttreatment performance on neuropsychological testing. Attention/processing speed improved on Digit Span, Spatial Span, PASAT, and Trail Making. Distractibility on list learning during and following the second list showed significant improvement. Memory improved on list learning for immediate and 30 minute delayed conditions. Reasoning improved slightly on Comprehension and dramatically on Similarities.

When he entered treatment, he reported that his deficits negatively impacted his work by as much as 50%. Following treatment he reported that his boss was pleased with his work and the patient felt that the negative impact on his work was dramatically reduced. He and his wife felt that he was functioning in all areas far better than he had been prior to treatment. They also agreed that while he was not functioning as well as he had been prior to the surgery, he was close to that level and far better than he had been for the previous 9 years.

Another case, RU, developed intractable seizures at age four and had significant learning problems throughout school. At age 33 he had a partial left temporal lobectomy. Frequency of partial complex seizures dropped from 1 or 2 per month

	Pretreatment (8 years postsurgery)	Posttreatment (9.5 yrs post)
Table 6.2 Changes in attention/information processing, memory, and intellectual functioning in RF, age 45		
WAIS III		
Digits forward	6 Digits	7 Digits
Digits backward	5 Digits	6 Digits
Comprehension (SS)	9	10
Similarities (SS)	10	17
WMS III		
Spatial span forward	5 Blocks	6 Blocks
Spatial span backward	4 Blocks	4 Blocks
Trails A	−0.5 SD	Average
Trails B	−1.6 SD	−0.4 SD
PASAT	Below AV/impaired	AV/above
CVLT/AVLT		
First trial	7/16	7/15
Fifth trial	12/16	15/15
Distraction list	4/16	9/15
Post distraction recall	62%	93%
30 minutes delay	10/16	14/15

to 1 or 2 per year. At this point he moved out of his parents' house and into an Epilepsy Foundation sponsored house. He took classes and placement exams for the GED. He was concurrently treated for depression with medication and psychotherapy. He nonetheless failed on two separate occasions to pass all parts of the GED. At this point he sought cognitive remediation.

Neuropsychological testing revealed attention, processing speed and memory were impaired. Trails A was below the 10th percentile. Trails B was within normal limits (35th percentile). List learning on the Memory Assessment Scales (MAS; 12 words)) was 38 words, cued recall was nine words, and list recognition was 11 words. FAS was at the 50th percentile.

Alternating attention (set shifting), processing speed and complex mental tracking on *Two in One* Level 3 is shown in Fig. 6.40. At baseline he was four standard deviations below the normative sample. He did even worse over the first two training trials. However, thereafter he was able to show substantial improvement (two standard deviations below normal.) Processing speed and ability to shift set on *Run Silent* Level 3 improved from a 55% hit rate to almost 80% (see Online Resource 16).

Memory strategies for verbal material were taught on *Memory Game* Level 2. The first month of training yielded an average of 35 words retained from the list whereas by the end of the second month he had almost doubled his performance (see Fig. 6.41). Memory strategies for nonverbal material were addressed on *Symbol Memory*. His average performance on session 1 was under 60% correct recall of the symbols. However, he recalled an average of 90% by the end of the second session.

At this point repeat neuropsychological testing was undertaken. Attention training seemed to have helped on Trails A and B (see Fig. 6.42). Trails A improved

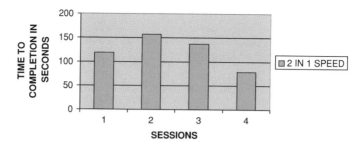

Fig. 6.40 RU alternating attention/complex mental tracking: Two in One level 3

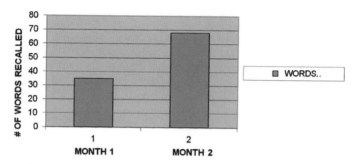

Fig. 6.41 RU verbal memory: Memory Game 2

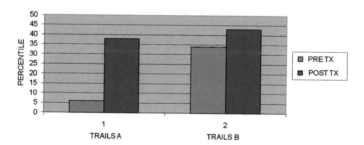

Fig. 6.42 RU attention, tracking and impulse control: Trail Making

to the normal level. Trails B improved, suggesting transfer of training or generalization from the set-shifting exercises practiced during treatment. Training in tracking, set-shifting, and impulse control (e.g., *Run Silent* 3, *Two in One* 3) seemed to have positively impacted his FAS score, which improved to the 80th percentile. List learning, cued recall, and recognition showed only modest improvement (Online Resources 17–19). However, it should be pointed out that there was a definite ceiling effect for recognition (i.e., 11 of 12 recognized pretreatment versus 12 out of 12 posttreatment).

There were several important life changes that took place as a consequence of treatment. First, he moved out of the Epilepsy Foundation sponsored apartment and found his own apartment in the community. He passed the GED exam. He began to attend a community college and took three courses in his first semester. He passed two of these and got an incomplete on the third because he had not completed all of the assignments. He subsequently did so and passed this course as well. He continued to attend an epilepsy support group and was contracted to create the logo for the newsletter and sweatshirts, as art and cartooning was his field of interest and study. He then entered into a business arrangement as a partner for a new start-up company.

Neurosurgical Symptoms and Mechanisms

Neurosurgery can obviously impact any number of cognitive domains, depending on the site of the intervention. Patients frequently do not recover fully from the effects of this invasive procedure. Cognitive symptoms from surgery may not differ from those produced by other etiologies and they respond well to cognitive remediation. Various regions of the brain may be temporarily or permanently impaired and some important areas may be cut in order to successfully complete the intervention. The nature of the symptoms and the etiology will determine whether compensatory mechanisms may be available for attempts at remediation.

Subcortical Disorders

CG was a 55-year-old woman who is a retired accountant. About four-and-a-half years before her referral for testing she developed motor dyscontrol, balance problems, and cognitive processing difficulty. She was worked up for multiple sclerosis (MS) and other subcortical diseases, but failed to meet the criteria for any of these diagnoses, although her symptoms were most similar to MS. She was felt to have an atypical subcortical disease.

Testing revealed mild to moderate cognitive impairment. Processing speed was mildly impaired and accuracy was borderline normal. Full Scale IQ was estimated to be above average. Immediate verbal memory and list learning were unimpaired but she demonstrated considerable perseveration on these tasks. Immediate visual–nonverbal memory was above average. She evidenced sustained attention problems when there was an executive functions component to the task.

Attention problems and perseveration were evidenced on *Get Q*, *Two in One* and *Dartboard* so these were included in her treatment plan. *Dartboard and Invaders* were included to help with her perceptual and spatial difficulties and *Double Trouble* was added to help with multitasking.

Performance on *Get Q* Level 1, which requires focused attention, was accurate but slow. Speed increased slowly and slightly over the first few sessions, but less

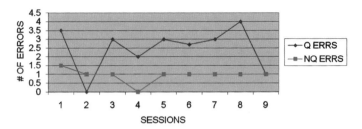

Fig. 6.43 CG alternating attention, impulse control and perceptual accuracy: errors on Get Q 3

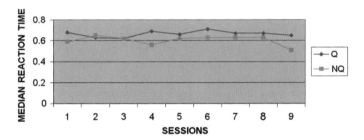

Fig. 6.44 CG alternating attention, impulse control, and perceptual accuracy: reaction time on Get Q 3

than usually seen in patients treated with NeurXercise. She then began to experiment with a treatment she had seen on TV that purportedly helped patients with MS. This involved controlled bee stings, the body's reaction to which purportedly reduced MS symptoms. Her motor and processing speed increased almost immediately. She continued to show improved performance within and between sessions, at a level similar to that seen with most patients. Online Resource 20 reflects that her accuracy was always within normal limits over nine sessions on *Get Q* Level 2. Alternating attention speed was normal (below 0.60 seconds) for Q and non-Q targets in two of the last three sessions (see Online Resource 21). *Get Q* 3 added more of a perceptual and impulse-control demand while performing essentially the same alternating attention task as *Get Q* 2. Figures 6.43 and 6.44 reflect that she was able to perform the task accurately and at the same reaction time as *Get Q* 2 for non-Q stimuli but she was a little slower on Q stimuli.

Alternating attention training continued on Level 2 of *Two in One*. She was highly variable in her accuracy, but was within normal limits on the last six trials (see Online Resource 22). Speed was excellent (only one session fell below the mean obtained by a normal sample). By the end of the training on Level 2 she was responding two standard deviations above the mean (see Online Resource 23). Levels 3 and 4 of *Two in One* added a mental manipulation component to the Level 2 task. Thus, spatial and executive functions were required in addition to alternating attention. Her performance on Levels 3 and 4 are depicted in Online Resources 24 and 25. Except for the first trial, all trials were within normal limits

Table 6.3 Changes in attention, memory, compensation, impairment, processing speed, and IQ in CG

Luria-Nebraska (CL = 54)					
R H Y	M E M	E L E V	I M P	S P D	I Q
55 Mo post onset	35	36	38	54	61	115
64 Mo post onset	31	43	41	42	52	122

for accuracy on Level 3. Similarly, she completed the task within a normal time frame, except for that first trial. Shifting to Level 4 to ensure that she was practicing the mental task and not responding to overlearned and memorized answers revealed that she was indeed performing the functions. The first trial was about one standard deviation below the mean but all subsequent trials were one to two standard deviations above the mean.

Continuing with visual spatial demands but now within the context of a sustained attention task, she reached the criterion by session four of *Dartboard* 2 and sustained this level of performance until the task was discontinued after session seven (see Online Resource 26). A visual spatial task that required sustained attention, rapid processing, and planning ahead was *Invaders* 3. Online Resource 27 demonstrates that she sustained her attention for a brief time (6 stimuli) on the first session and earned 360 points on average. However, by the end of training she was sustaining her attention for more than 40 stimuli and averaged more than 100 points higher than her initial score.

Multitasking was practiced on *Double Trouble*, an exercise that requires the simultaneous performance of two visual motor tasks. She practiced four trials with the criterion set at 600 points. By trial three she obtained an average score on one of the two tasks and by trial four she was above average on both tasks (see Online Resource 28). The criterion was then increased to 1,000 points. She performed within the average range on both tasks for three consecutive trials (see Online Resource 29). The criterion was then raised to 2,000 points. She continued with the same level of success over this increased amount of time (see Online Resource 30). When the second task to be completed was changed (Level 2), there was no change in her ability to master two tasks simultaneously (see Online Resource 31). In fact, she maintained excellent accuracy on one task (average score per rocket launched exceeded 90) while performing near or at the very best obtainable performance on the second task. She was then shifted back to level 1 and she demonstrated a continued high level of divided attention (see Online Resource 32).

Posttreatment neuropsychological testing revealed increase in measured IQ from above average to superior (Table 6.3). Motor and processing speed on the same table improved from mildly impaired to within normal limits and overall brain impairment improved from borderline impaired to well within normal limits

Table 6.4 Changes in attention, processing speed, and executive functioning on PASAT in CG

PASAT errors (levin modification)					
55 Mo post onset	12	17	23	32	84 (−1.3 SD)
64 Mo post onset	3	14	23	30	70 (+1.2 SD)

Table 6.5 Changes in visual scanning, attention, and set-shifting on trail making on CG

	Trail making test	
	A	B
55 MO post onset	47 s	83 s
	−1 SD	−0.25 SD
64 MO post onset	29 s	78 s
	+0.5 SD	AV

($p < 0.01$). There were no significant improvements or decrements on LNNB measures of attention (C2), memory (C10), or compensation (S4), all of which were within normal limits prior to treatment onset. Processing speed improved on PASAT and Trails A (Tables 6.4 and 6.5). Total PASAT errors were 1.3 standard deviations below average prior to intervention but 1.2 standard deviations above average following intervention (an improvement of 2.5 standard deviations). Trails A was 0.5 standard deviations below average before treatment but was average posttreatment, compared to normals given a second administration of the test (i.e., practice effects were controlled by using norms for repeated administrations).

Executive functioning was normal and unchanged on Trails B (Table 6.5). Divided attention on Trigrams dropped from above average to average. Amount of perseveration on AVLT (Table 6.6) dropped dramatically on posttreatment testing, from nine perseverations to none. There were no interference effects before or after treatment on AVLT (Table 6.6) in that Trial 1 and B list performance were both average and she had perfect recall after the distracter list (i.e., short delay condition) on both occasions. Thus, AVLT perseverations was the only executive function measure that was outside of the normal range prior to treatment and it improved dramatically following treatment.

Verbal memory and list learning on AVLT was initially impaired on trial 2. Following training, all trials were at or above normal performance (see Table 6.6). It appeared that learning was slowed on the first two trials but thereafter she had no difficulty, even before treatment. Delays of 30 minutes did not reduce her recall and recognition before or after treatment (see Table 6.6). Thus, initial list learning but not retention or retrieval were initial problems. Initial learning was no longer a problem after treatment, suggesting that remediating attention addressed the underlying cause of her learning problem.

She reported several impressive changes in her life following treatment. Her success on the exercises and in daily functioning improved her self-esteem and self-confidence. She reported successfully pursuing her writing, which had ceased due to her symptoms. She reported more energy and motor control. She felt that her thinking speed was back to premorbid levels.

Table 6.6 Changes in memory, learning, and executive functioning on AVLT in CG

	1	2	3	4	5	B	I R	D R	D R G	P S V
55 Mo post onset	9	11	14	15	14	9	15	15	15	9
64 Mo post onset	7	11	14	15	15	7	15	15	15	0

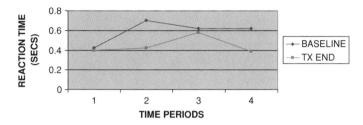

Fig. 6.45 MS processing speed on Get Q (level 1)

Another case of subcortical disorder was MS, a 43-year-old computer pro-grammer who was diagnosed with multiple sclerosis 19 months prior to receiving neuropsychological testing. His ambulation was assisted by the use of a cane. Processing speed was in the low end of the average range on the WMS III and impaired on PASAT. Immediate and delayed memory were average for stories, faces, family pictures, and verbal paired associates. However, this seemed below expected premorbid functioning in light of education and occupation. The Beck Depression Inventory was in the mildly depressed range.

Processing speed was practiced on *Get Q* 1 and *Two in One* Levels 1, 2 and 3. Figure 6.45 reflects that after the first minute or so, his ability to quickly process the data is lost on *Get Q* 1. During the first quarter of the task his reaction time is normal but becomes mildly impaired thereafter. With training he maintained normal processing speed and reaction times throughout the entire exercise. Baseline processing speed on *Two in One* was one standard deviation below average on Levels 1 and 3 and two standard deviations below average on Level 2. Figure 6.46 reveals that processing speed improved to about one standard devia-tion above average on Levels 1 and 2, and about two standard deviations above average on Level 3. Divided attention places considerable emphasis on processing speed so *Double Trouble* was added to his training regimen. Online Resource 33 reflects that on Level 1 he started out with 25% accuracy on rockets and 50% accuracy in responding to letters at the same time. However, he completed the training at 90% accuracy for rockets and 100% accurate responding to the letters. On Level 2 he began with 60% accuracy on the rockets but at a cost of missing all notes. By the end of treatment he responded with 100% accuracy to both rockets and notes (see Online Resource 34).

Memory training involved *Memory Game* 2, *Symbol Memory* and *Line Up* 3. Online Resource 35 demonstrates that he remembered 30% of the words on

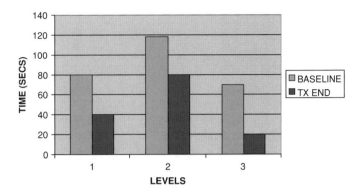

Fig. 6.46 MS processing speed-2 in 1

Table 6.7 Changes in attention/distractibility, memory, and depression in MS, age 43	Pretreatment (19 months post diagnosis)	Posttreatment (40 months post)
PASAT (% errors)	57	37
WMS III		
Processing speed index	93	99
Logical mem (I/II)	9/10	12/13
Verbal paired assoc (I/II)	9/10	13/13
Faces (I/II)	11/13	9/12
Family pictures (I/II)	9/9	10/11
Beck depression inventory	14	27

Memory Game 2 at baseline but 95% of the words by the end of treatment. His recall of symbols at baseline was 50% but reached 97% by the end of training (Online Resource 36). Similarly, facial recognition on *Line Up* 3 improved from 55% accuracy to 95%. At this point repeat testing was undertaken.

In terms of processing speed (Table 6.7) the percentage of PASAT errors was calculated because two different versions of the test were used to reduce practice effects. He improved from 57% errors to 37% errors. On WMS III the Processing Speed Index improved from 93 to 99. These appeared to represent consistent, modest improvement in an area frequently associated with MS deficit and disability (Christodoulou 2005; Denney et al. 2005). Further, neuropsychological testing studies of MS patients (Filley et al. 1990; Julian 2007) have found a steady downward trend. This suggested that benefit derived may be much greater than it at first appeared. At the very least, he did not become more impaired on the tests as his cohort did.

Similar to processing speed, Christodoulou (2005) reports that learning and recall of information are typically impaired in patients with MS and Filley et al. (1990) observed a downward trend in memory functioning. However, with treatment, the patient improved in this area. Table 6.7 reveals that verbal memory improved from average to above average on stories and paired associates. Facial memory did not improve over baseline and may represent a statistically insignificant decrease on one measure and a similarly insignificant increase on the other. The final scores on the table reflected that he had become more depressed over the course of treatment although he showed improvement or lack of significant decline on neuropsychological testing.

At termination he reported greater efficiency at work. He also started his own computer consulting business. There are several factors that support the conclusion that cognitive changes on testing and behavioral improvement in daily functioning were likely due to the intervention. First, his steroid dosage had remained constant throughout treatment so it could not account for the changes. Second, spontaneous recovery or improvement would not be expected 2 years following his being diagnosed. Third, when compared to individuals similarly diagnosed with MS of the exacerbation-remission type who were his age, he showed improvement or no change over the same elapsed time period that they declined. Lastly, his depression worsened from mild to moderate/severe on the Beck, which suggested that emotional issues were not a major contributor to his cognitive problems or improvement. This leaves cognitive remediation as the most likely cause for his improved level of functioning. These positive effects of cognitive remediation with an MS patient are similar to those obtained in a case report by Caruso and Ash (2007) who used a similar cognitive remediation approach developing compensatory and restorative strategies.

The case of RB involved subcortical damage caused by head trauma. RB was a 21-year-old high school educated man who worked in the military honor guard until he was in an automobile accident that resulted in a moderate brain injury. He had a brief loss of consciousness and a posttraumatic amnesia of 12 hours. MRI revealed hemorrhage of the left precentral paramedian subcortex. He was treated in a brain rehabilitation program and 1 year later follow-up neuropsychological testing revealed residual attentional problems and mild dysphoria. He also suffered back and knee injuries from the accident. His assignment was changed from the prestigious honor guard to "helper" in a clinic, which usually entailed answering phones, running errands, and covering for people when they went to lunch.

Two years post injury he was again tested and found to have residual attention, learning, and memory problems. His job remained "helper" in the clinic. At this point cognitive remediation was initiated. Attention and executive functioning were targeted while learning and memory were not addressed in order to determine whether attentional deficits accounted for the problems in these other areas.

Focused and sustained attention were practiced over the course of three sessions on Level 1 of *Get Q*. Response time improved from impaired to normal (see Fig. 6.47). Speed of sustained and alternating attention on *Get Q* 2 improved from impaired to normal over the course of three sessions (see Fig. 6.48). Accuracy remained unimpaired over all sessions. Generalization of training in sustained and alternating attention was seen in his performance on *Two in One* in which criterion was reached in only three trials within a single session. This was true for Level 1, in which accuracy was good and speed improved to normal (see Fig. 6.49) and Level 2, in which speed and accuracy improved to normal over three trials within a single session (see Fig. 6.50).

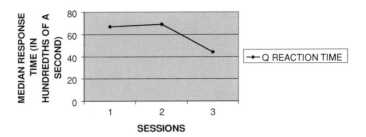

Fig. 6.47   RB focused and sustained attention: Get Q 1

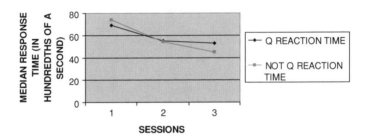

Fig. 6.48   RB sustained and alternating attention: Get Q 2 speed

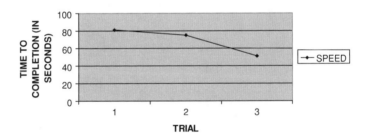

Fig. 6.49   RB sustained and alternating attention: speed on Two in One level 1

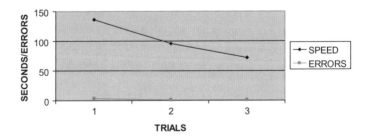

Fig. 6.50   RB sustained and alternating attention: Two in One 2

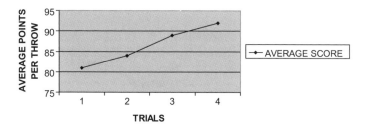

Fig. 6.51 RB sustained attention: Dartboard 2 (1,000 pts)

Ability to sustain attention for increasing periods of time was practiced on *Dartboard* Level 2. It took four trials to reach criterion (averaging over 89 points per throw) when the goal was 1,000 points (about 1 minute of sustained attention). These results are depicted in Fig. 6.51. When the demand was raised to about 10 minutes of sustained attention, he was able to exceed an average of 89 points for seven consecutive trials (see Online Resource 37).

Executive functions were next addressed. Set shifting on Level 3 of *Run Silent* was improved to at least 90% accuracy on both alternating trajectories by the fifth practice trial and continued at this level of accuracy on the sixth trial (see Online Resource 38). Rapid set shifting on *Run Silent* 4 was accomplished in five practice sessions (see Online Resource 39). On this task height and depth of plane and submarine shift on every trial.

Multitasking was practiced on *Double Trouble*. On Level 1 over three trials he was able to maintain approximately 80% accuracy on one task while performing optimally on another task presented simultaneously (see Online Resource 40). On Level 2 the time spent practicing divided attention was increased tenfold. Four of the five trials were performed within the preset criterion of over 90% accuracy for notes and an average in excess of 89 fuel units gathered per rocket (see Online Resource 41). A third task was then introduced so that he performed the same two tasks for the same extended period (about 10 minutes) while reciting names within a category (e.g., cities, countries, women's names, men's names, manufactured items, etc.) Online Resource 42 demonstrates that the introduction of the third task led to deterioration of performance on the first trial but that he maintained criterion performance for the following nine trials.

Set shifting within a problem solving task was practiced on *Mission Decode* and *Detective*. On Level 1 of *Mission Decode* he failed less than halfway through the task. However, on the second attempt he passed the task with only one error (see Online Resource 43). On the more complex *Mission Decode* 2 he failed on his first two attempts but passed on his next three, improving from four errors on trials three and four to three errors on trial 5 (see Online Resource 44). He had no difficulty passing the first level of *Detective* on his first attempt. On the second level he made three errors on his first two attempts and had a perfect score on the third trial (see Online Resource 45). Practice on *Mission Decode* seemed to have

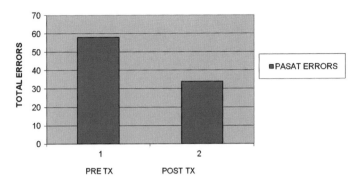

Fig. 6.52 RB PASAT performance

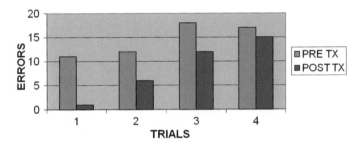

Fig. 6.53 RB PASAT errors

generalized as reflected in improved performance on the set shifting-problem solving tasks on *Detective*.

At this point his treatment was felt to be complete and retesting was undertaken. Sustained auditory verbal attention on PASAT improved from the 37th percentile to the 70th percentile (see Fig. 6.52). Performance on each trial of PASAT is shown in Fig. 6.53. Pretreatment scores ranged from 26th to 58th percentile while posttreatment scores were 53rd to 78th percentile. Sustained attention for visual–nonverbal material on the 1990s version of ANAM improved from impaired to normal for a 5 minute period. Accuracy improved from almost four standard deviations below normal to one standard deviation above normal while efficiency improved from about 0.2 standard deviations below the mean to about 0.3 standard deviations above the mean. Results on the Trail Making Test appear in Fig. 6.54. Visual scanning and attention on Trails A improved from the 48th percentile to the 81st percentile. Alternating visual attention on Trails B improved from the 59th percentile to the 89th percentile. Thus, attention showed significant improvement following remediation.

Set shifting is an executive function. It showed dramatic improvement on Trails B and PASAT, as cited above.

List learning improved on AVLT from the 5th percentile to the 46th percentile. Memory under distraction conditions remained impaired (LIST B

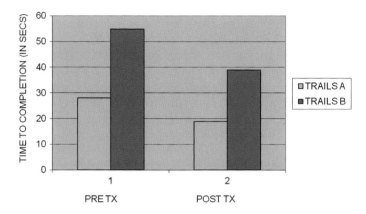

Fig. 6.54 RB trail making test performance

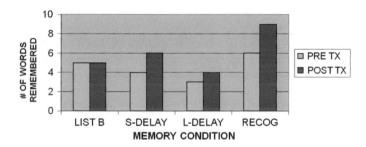

Fig. 6.55 RB AVLT memory performance

remained at 19th percentile and Short-Delay went from 1st percentile to 2nd percentile, see Fig. 6.55). Delayed memory after 30 minutes was likewise impaired and unchanged (<1st percentile to 1st percentile for recall and < 1st percentile to 4th percentile for recognition, see Fig. 6.55). After delays of 15 minutes, recall was still impaired on LNNB for tactile memory and a seven-word list (he remembered two of seven words after treatment compared to one of seven words before treatment).

Learning deficits may have been due to attentional problems as they seem to have improved following remediation. However, memory problems remained, suggesting that attention was not the underlying cause of the memory deficits and that they would need to be addressed independently if he were to improve in this area. The retesting suggested that significant improvement occurred in the areas treated but that no meaningful improvement occurred in the untreated area.

He reported that he was liked at work and they were pleased with his performance. He no longer got irritated and angry with the staff or the job, although this was a problem in the early phases of treatment. Perhaps, improvement in this area was due to enhanced self-esteem as he saw his functioning improve.

Subcortical Symptoms and Mechanisms

As can readily be seen from the above cases of subcortical disorder, the areas of balance, motor strength and control, processing speed, and attention are most likely to be affected and not show spontaneous recovery. Executive functions and many types of memory rely on higher cognitive abilities mediated by cortical regions and therefore tend to be less affected and more easily remediated when they are found in subcortical disorders. Depression, irritability/explosiveness, and self-esteem/self-image issues are common in this group. This may be due to disruption in the limbic system, amygdala–hippocampal complex dysfunction, and/or psychological response to cognitive and behavioral deficits.

Co-morbid Conditions

KP was a 65-year-old gentleman who worked as a scientist. A few years before he was evaluated, he had two carotid endocarderectomies that resulted in a left hemisphere stroke. He was also diagnosed with mitral valve prolapse, insulin-dependent diabetes, hypertension, peripheral vascular disease, and hypercholesterolemia (high cholesterol).

He was taking 11 different medications for these conditions. He felt that he had problems with memory, judgment, and confusion/distractibility. Working memory was average while other WAIS III composite scores were above average. He had difficulty with visual processing speed, set shifting, distractibility, initial learning, and divided attention.

Attention, visual processing speed, and distractibility are inherent in the exercises *Get Q* Levels 1 and 2 and *Dartboard* Level 2. His baseline scores were below average on *Get Q* 1 and highly variable on *Get Q* 2 so these exercises were included in his treatment plan. His average was below 80 points per throw on *Dartboard* so this too was added to the treatment plan. The same cognitive skills plus set shifting are inherent in *Two in One*. Baseline scores on all levels of *Two in One* were impaired for speed and accuracy so this was added to the treatment plan. *Line Up* Level 3 was used for training facial memory. Executive functions were practiced on *Mission Decode*, a problem solving-set shifting exercise, *Detective*, and *Number Guesser* 2, as well as *Two in One* above.

On *Get Q* 1 he was able to bring his speed into the normal range on two consecutive sessions spaced 1 week apart (Online Resource 46). Accuracy was within normal limits on all trials. On *Get Q* Level 2 he showed steady improvement from session 3 through session 6 when his speed and accuracy reached the normal range (Online Resources 47 and 48). Online Resource 49 depicts performance on the last trial of sessions 1 and 2 of *Two in One* 1. By the end of session 2 accuracy and speed were within normal limits. Similarly, on *Two in One* 2, which introduced an additional impulse control element, he finished the first session about one standard deviation below normal and finished the second session within normal limits for both speed and accuracy (Online Resource 50). On Two in One 3/4, which required mental arithmetic to complete the alternating attention task, he completed the first session about two standard deviations slower than the norm. However, by the end of the second session his speed was only slightly slower than the norm (less than a standard deviation below the mean; see Online Resource 51) and accuracy was within normal limits (Online Resource 52). By the end of the third session speed was at the mean of the normal group and he committed no errors (Online Resources 51 and 52).

He practiced 17–19 trials per session on Dartboard Level 2. Online Resource 53 demonstrates a steady improvement over three sessions. He met the criterion of at least two consecutive trials of 90 points or higher. In fact, the last three trials of session 3 all exceeded 90 points per throw over the course of reaching 2,000 points at a speed set to 10.

We then turned to remediating his memory deficits. Initially, he had difficulty with Memory Game 2. He was instructed in compensatory strategies using the auditory mode. His best performance during session 1 was 23 correct out of 31 words. However, on session 2 he got 58 out of 58 words. He practiced the strategies on Shopping List and was eventually able to get 37 of the 39 items. Facial memory on Line Up Level 3 (Online Resource 54) improved from a baseline of 12 correct (60% accuracy) to 19 correct (95% accuracy) over three practice sessions. Memorization was not an issue as the target faces changed on each trial and the response choices were different poses of the target individual and people with common features to the target.

Executive functions of reasoning, judgment, and set shifting were addressed with Detective. On Level 1 he identified the correct analogy 19 out of 21 times whereas his baseline had been 13 (see Online Resource 55). He had no difficulty with the verbal analog (24 out of 25 compared to a baseline of 19; see Online Resource 55), suggesting that the previous set shifting exercises (e.g., *Get Q* 2, *Two in One* 1, 2, 3 and 4) had led to generalization and remediation of set shifting. The next executive functioning exercise attempted was *Mission Decode*, a problem solving and set-shifting task (Online Resource 56). At baseline, he "blew up" after 35 problems on the simplest level (29 correct answers and 6 errors) whereas following set shifting training, he completed the task without "blowing up" (60 of 64 problems correctly solved). He "blew up" after he solved 34 of the 40 problems (85% correct) on the most difficult level. That is, he solved 34 of the 39 he had seen and there were a total of 40 problems comprising the exercise. *Number Guesser* Level 2, which required hypothesis generation and use of feedback was the last executive function task. His score was highly variable throughout the exercise but never outside of the criterion for successful performance set forth in the NeurXercise manual.

Repeat neuropsychological testing reflected improvement in verbal learning, memory, and freedom from distractibility. No change was noted in executive functioning on the tests. Figure 6.56 demonstrates that his initial performance in verbal learning was poor prior to remediation but improved significantly following

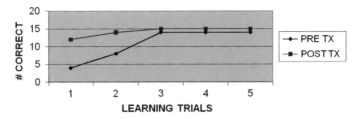

Fig. 6.56 KP verbal learning and memory: AVLT performance

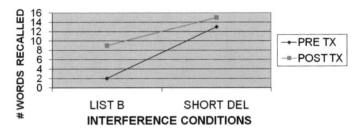

Fig. 6.57 KP interference effects: AVLT performance

treatment. At baseline his best performance was 14 of 15 words learned and remembered whereas at posttreatment he maintained perfect performance on the last three trials (15 out of 15). Proactive interference was seen prior to treatment (compare Fig. 6.57 trial 1 in pretreatment with Fig. 6.57 List B in pretreatment) in which he lost 50% of his learning capacity after five practice trials were followed by a new list (4 words remembered on trial 1 of the first list versus 2 words remembered on presentation of a second list). There was much less proactive inhibition following treatment (the interference effect is 25%–12 words remembered versus nine words, which was still normal performance). Retroactive interference was measured by the short delay condition on AVLT. After learning 14 of the 15 words at baseline, interference caused the loss of one of those words (13 words remembered after interference). Following treatment, he learned all 15 words and retained them all after the interference. After 30 minutes he recalled and recognized all 15 words. Unfortunately, the 30 minute delay was not given at pretreatment baseline. However, since he never got all the words correct at pretreatment, this likely represented improvement.

Verbal processing speed improved modestly on the Golden version of the Stroop ($T = 29.5$ at baseline and $T = 37$ at posttreatment). Nonverbal processing speed on Stroop did not change ($T = 35.7$ versus $T = 36$).

No changes were found on tests of executive functions. Category Test performance was normal at baseline and posttreatment. PASAT was about 1.5 standard deviations below average on both occasions. The T was below 40 on each occasion for the Stroop Interference task.

Ecologically valid changes were observed. He and his wife felt he was attending, processing, and remembering better. He successfully made several speeches at scientific conventions. He appeared on a TV special with other scientists in his area of expertise and articulately discussed his theories and research (he provided me with a copy of the videotape). Finally, he applied for and received a research grant that had eluded him for years, even prior to his stroke.

Another complex case of co-morbid conditions was that of JP, a 34-year-old man who contracted Acute Lymphoblastic Leukemia at age 14. He developed leukoencephalopathy, secondary to radiation and chemotherapy. In addition, he developed Bells Palsy and Herpes Zoster/Shingles, secondary to medication treatment. At age 28 he developed spinal meningitis. He was placed in nursing homes and rehabilitation facilities over the next year-and-a-half and received Occupational, Physical, and Speech Therapies. He was responding to the treatments when he suddenly became lethargic and was diagnosed with Syndrome of Inappropriate Diuretic Hormone. He was placed in a nursing home for the next year. He then received an operation that improved his mental status. He improved over the next 3 years and was then referred for cognitive remediation to help with his impulsivity, attention, perceptual/spatial ability, and reasoning processes. The patient was wheelchair bound, had little motion in his hands and spoke breathily and inarticulately.

Baseline neuropsychological testing with the LNNB revealed significant overall brain impairment with little evidence of compensation. There were significant problems with manual motor skills, tactile perception, arithmetic calculations, memory, and intellectual processing. There was moderate impairment in the areas of visual perception, spatial abilities, receptive language, and reading. His scores were mildly impaired on focused auditory attention and expressive language. Impulsivity can be assessed qualitatively by counting the number of perseverations made during the administration of the battery. The cutoff for normal limits is set at three perseverations, as 95.8% of the normal group gave fewer than four perseverations. The patient produced seven perseverations, consistent with the complaints of his being impulsive.

All tasks required him to use the computer manually so it was expected that motor functioning would improve over the course of treatment, as he would be forced to use fine motor skills. His impulsivity was addressed with *Get Q* and *Two in One*. Memory training employed *Memory Game* 2, *Shopping List*, and *Symbol Memory*. Perceptual/spatial problems were treated with *Dartboard, Run Silent*, and *Invaders*. *Detective* and *Mission Decode* were used to help improve reasoning and executive functioning.

He was able to eventually meet the criteria for normal performance on most exercises. For example, alternating attention on *Run Silent* 3 eventually was performed at 83% accuracy for each trajectory and list learning was accurately performed on *Memory Game* 2 for seven of seven words. The exception was for impulsivity/perseverations on *Two in One* 2. As can be seen in Fig. 6.58, he improved dramatically by the third trial and met the criterion for normal performance on the sixth trial but could not maintain this level of performance on the

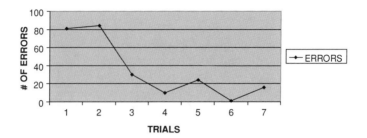

Fig. 6.58 JP impulsivity/perseveration and alternating attention: Two in One 2

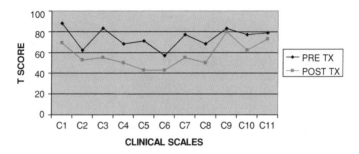

Fig. 6.59 JP performance on LNNB clinical scales

seventh trial. Most of his errors did not involve failure to shift set between numbers and letters but rather were due to impulsive responding or perseveration on number of key strokes (i.e., the number of key strokes for letters and numbers were equal between "AA11 and II99" but thereafter there were two letter strokes to four number strokes, "JJ1010", "KK1111", etc.).

Posttreatment testing revealed that the number of perseverations dropped from 7 to 1 on the LNNB. Figure 6.59 shows the dramatic improvement on the clinical scales of the LNNB following treatment. T scores below 59 were in the normal range (lower T scores were better on LNNB). Motor performance improvement was seen on C1 and C7. Writing on C7 returned to the normal range and both C1 and C7 showed significant improvement over baseline ($p < 0.01$). Auditory focused attention, measured by C2, returned to the normal range and was one T point from being significant at the 0.05 level. Attention and motor improvement likely accounted for significant change in tactile sensation ($p < 0.01$). Likewise, reading on C8 likely improved due to better attention. Visual perceptual training seemed to have been highly beneficial in light of the improvement to normal performance on C4, a change that was significant at $p < 0.01$. Receptive and expressive speech improvements were significant at $p < 0.01$, reflecting positive effects of speech therapy he had re-entered following improvement in his impulsive behavior. Immediate memory improved ($p < 0.01$). Reasoning, as measured by C11, improved to a nonsignificant degree and no change was noted in arithmetic, which was not addressed in the treatment plan. Since attention was clearly

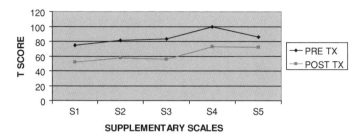

Fig. 6.60 JP performance on LNNB supplementary scales

improved, his arithmetic problems seemed not to be related to attention deficit. Figure 6.60 represents performance on the LNNB supplementary scales. All scales showed significant improvement ($p < 0.01$). S1 reflected that chronic deficits improved to normal levels. S4 reflected significant improvement in use of compensatory mechanisms, a key component of cognitive remediation. S5 reflected overall brain impairment improved from severe to moderate. S3 and S4 reflected bilateral sensorimotor improvement.

As mentioned above, his improved impulse control led to his return to speech therapy from which he had previously been terminated as having reached maximum medical benefit. His speech improved dramatically with additional speech therapy. He was likewise readmitted to physical therapy and benefited greatly. As his manual motor skills improved from using the computer, his mother began to teach him the piano. He was successful in this endeavor. His doctor and the nursing home staff insisted that he and his mother accept that he would remain wheelchair-bound for the rest of his life and not hold out impossible hopes to the contrary. His mother insisted on working with him on the use of a walker. After 1 week the nursing staff noted the amazing progress he was making and added use of a walker to his nursing care plan. Thereafter, staff and mother spent time working with him until he could use the walker regularly. Some time later he learned to ambulate with the use of two canes. While he had been told he could not function outside of the nursing home, he eventually moved into an assisted living apartment and had done well. He regularly visited his friends at the nursing home. Over the 5 years since he left treatment, he developed some psychiatric problems that included visual hallucinations. Thus, while cognitive remediation was helpful in many ways, there may be additional sequelae that require attention if patients are to return to "normal living".

Symptoms and Mechanisms in Co-morbid Conditions

With multiple, co-morbid conditions patients are better able to recover if the insults are consecutive and there is time to recover between neurological events. With multisystem problems, as is seen with KP, stability of the different conditions is essential for effective cognitive intervention. As long as there are areas of cognitive strength that can serve as a means of compensation, cognitive remediation can be helpful.

Cognitive Domain

Attention

MA was a high school graduate who fell from a moving vehicle and suffered a left-sided basilar skull fracture. He was hospitalized for 3 days. He had an anterograde amnesia for 1 week following the accident. There was a left-sided paralysis that resolved except for occasional episodes of palsy. His sense of smell and taste were impaired. He returned to work but he was overcome by gas fumes, which he had been unable to smell. Seven months post injury he was experiencing blackouts, headaches, and "twitching" on the left side. Audition and balance problems accompanied these episodes. CT was normal. He persisted having posttraumatic headaches, problems with memory, distraction, and visual perception, and met the DSM IV criteria for PTSD due to exaggerated startle response, flashbacks, palpitations, etc. whenever he rode as a passenger in a car.

Intellectual functioning was in the superior range. Executive functions were disrupted during visual tasks only. Sustained attention was impaired on visual tasks but not auditory ones. Encoding and retrieval of an auditorially presented word-list were mildly impaired while efficiency in learning the list was moderately to severely impaired. When there was a context, as opposed to a list of unrelated words, he performed well (e.g., a story, meaningful word-picture associations). His auditory verbal memory was disrupted by distraction, and verbal memory, in general, was mildly impaired on LNNB. Visual–nonverbal memory was intact. He performed normally on sensorimotor functions, focused attention, language, and visual perception.

He entered psychotherapy for PTSD, secondary to the accident, and cognitive remediation focused on his visual attention problems. At baseline, his major difficulties were on the most complex visual attention exercises, *Get Q* 3 (all letters are similarly shaped: Q, O, D, C, etc.), *Run Silent* 4 (height and depth change every trial) and *Double Trouble*. These constituted his treatment plan.

On *Get Q* 3 his accuracy was always within normal limits and speed improved from average to above average over three sessions (Fig. 6.61). He then began performing another task while working on *Get Q* 3, making it a divided attention task as well as a sustained and alternating attention task. While practicing *Get Q* 3, he also generated names of countries, models of cars, words beginning with designated letters, different sports, cities, articles of clothing, etc. As can be seen in Fig. 6.62 his performance slowed on the first trial but was back to normal speed compared with norms for the simpler *Get Q* 2 by itself (0.50–0.0.60 seconds for Q

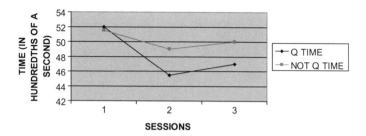

Fig. 6.61 MA sustained visual and alternating attention: Get Q level 3

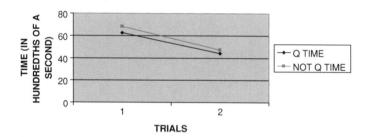

Fig. 6.62 MA sustained/alternating/divided attention: Get Q level 3 + additional task

and 0.44–0.62 seconds for not Q; median normative score is 0.56 seconds for both Q and not Q). Errors always remained within the limits seen on the simpler *Get Q* 2. This practice on divided attention generalized to *Double Trouble* on which he had no errors on Level 1 and only one error on Level 2.

On *Run Silent* Level 4 submarine and plane fire alternately and their projectiles have different trajectories (thus requiring alternating attention). In addition, the crafts change depth and height on each trial (set shifting, impulse control, and recalibrating are executive functions involved on this visuospatial-motor task). He was able to perform the task with a total of one miss after five trials. While there are no norms collected for this complex task, on the simpler *Run Silent* 3, which does not vary height and depth, normals initially have an average of ten misses. At this point his treatment was felt to be complete and neuropsychological testing was repeated.

Visual sustained attention improved to average for accuracy and above average for efficiency on Running Memory from the 1990s ANAM Battery (86.79–97.48 for accuracy and 83.02–119.72 for efficiency). Trails A improved to average. Thus, visual sustained attention was no longer impaired, as measured by repeat testing. Similarly, Trails B returned to average, suggesting visual alternating attention was no longer impaired. Regarding word-list performance, his total words learned over five trials improved more than a full standard deviation on AVLT. His retention by the fifth trial returned to average from 0.75 standard deviations below the mean at baseline. His verbal learning under interference and in general improved to no errors on LNNB. Thus, verbal learning and memory showed significant improvement with attention training only, suggesting that attention problems were the root cause of much of his memory difficulty.

Following treatment he got a job in the maintenance department of a manufacturing company and enrolled in a college engineering program. He completed an Associates degree in Mechanical and Electrical Engineering and moved into the engineering department of the company for which he had been working. He worked as a manufacturing engineer and controlling engineer, with duties that included quality assurance and insuring production capability increases. Five years posttreatment he was in his final semester of completing his Bachelor of Science in Electromechanical Engineering Science. He was happily married and raising a family. He enjoyed a good relationship with his family of origin. His major continuing problem was an explosive temper. He sought treatment for this after terminating cognitive remediation, but was given a variety of medications with side effects worse than the symptoms they were prescribed to treat. He felt no one had followed him carefully or consistently and he discontinued medication and follow-up. It was recommended that he seek behavioral and psychological help from a psychologist or neuropsychologist who understood about emotional sequelae to head injuries and could help determine whether medication were appropriate during the course of psychotherapeutic follow-up.

HJ was a 23-year-old high school educated mechanic in the military. He suffered a closed head injury while overseas. He had a loss of consciousness for an undetermined period and required oxygen while in the hospital. He was transferred to an overseas military hospital and then returned to the States. A few months later he had a fall. Toward the end of the acute phase of his injury he was tested and found to be suffering from attention, verbal memory, language, and executive functioning problems. He was re-examined 6 months later. Memory had improved but the other areas had not. He entered a research project aimed at remediating attention problems. His scores on this second testing will be compared to his performance following treatment.

Sustained and alternating attention were addressed by NeurXercise. Baseline performance was below expectation on *Get Q* 2, *Two in One* 1 and 3/4, *Type It* 2 and 3, and *Dartboard* 2. Divided attention was below expectation for *Double Trouble* 1 and 2. These exercises became his treatment plan. Online Resource 57 reflects that he took seven sessions on *Get Q* 2 to bring his error rate consistently into normal limits while responding within normal speeds. It took only six sessions to complete *Two in One* on Level 1 such that speed and accuracy were consistently within the normal range (Online Resource 58). On *Two in One* Levels 3 and 4, Fig. 6.63 plots his baseline under trial block 1 while blocks 2–5 are the means for blocks of four trials. Accuracy was excellent on the last three blocks of four trials and speed was within normal limits on blocks three and five. *Type It* Level 2 improved from four errors to two in only one trial (Online Resource 59). On Level 3 of *Type It* he improved from a baseline of six errors to only one error after only two trials. He raised his *Dartboard* performance in just two trials from an average of 80 points to the goal of exceeding 89 points per throw (Online Resource 60).

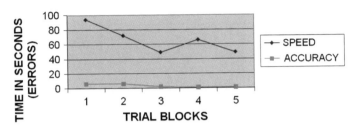

Fig. 6.63 HG sustained and alternating attention: Two in One level ¾

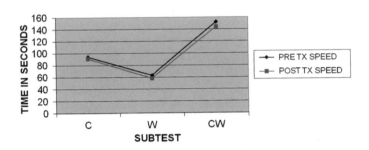

Fig. 6.64 HJ time to complete Stroop

He began working on divided attention by practicing *Double Trouble* Level 1 for a goal of 600 points on one exercise and accurate letter responses on the other. The task took about a minute. He was able to consistently be accurate on both tasks by trials 5 and 6 (Online Resource 61). Both of these tasks were visual, but one was verbal and the other was not. He next worked on Level 2 in which both tasks are nonverbal, but one is visual and the other auditory. The goal remained 600 points and accurate responding to the stimuli. He reached the goal consistently by trial 8 (Online Resource 62). The task length was then increased by raising the goal to 1,500 points (2–3 minutes for task duration). Consistency was maintained at the desired level by trial 12. The task length was then further increased by raising the goal to 3,000 points (4–5 minutes of sustained attention). He maintained normal performance for both trials administered (Online Resource 63). He was then administered Level 1 again (Online Resource 64) but at a goal of 3,000 points (4–5 minutes of sustained attention). Except for the first trial, he scored at the goal of at least 90% accuracy of letters and an average of at least 90 points per throw. The task was repeated at the same level but a third task was introduced (counting by ones while performing the two visual-motor computer tasks.) By trial 6 he was performing at the same level as he had during the two-task exercise (Online Resource 65).

Figures 6.64 and 6.65 reflect that on the Kaplan version of the Stroop there was no significant change for speed on visual–nonverbal material (naming the colors of the blocks) but that accuracy improved by more than four standard deviations, from very impaired to normal. Verbal speed improved about 0.7 standard deviations while accuracy with verbal material improved from two standard deviations

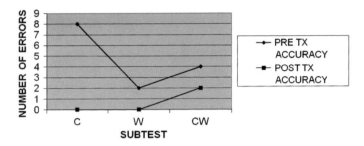

Fig. 6.65 HJ accuracy on Stroop

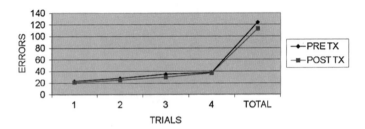

Fig. 6.66 HJ PASAT performance

below average to normal (no errors). Speed on the executive functions task of the Stroop improved a full standard deviation, from approximately −1.5 standard deviations from the mean to about −0.5 standard deviations from the mean. Accuracy improved from slightly below the mean to 0.5 standard deviations above the mean. Thus, on the Stroop there is clear improvement in his accuracy and mixed results regarding improvement in speed.

Simple visual tracking speed on Trails A remained in the normal range while speed of alternating attention on Trails B remained impaired at approximately the same level (−3 standard deviations). Consistent, although statistically nonsignificant, improvement was evident at all presentation speeds on the PASAT (Fig. 6.66). Total errors improved about a half standard deviation. Sustained attention on the 1990s ANAM Running Memory was measured by administering the test twice consecutively so that the second score represented sustained attention over a 10 minutes period (5 minutes of practice followed by a second 5 minute trial). On the second administration he scored almost three standard deviations below the norm for accuracy prior to treatment but improved to 0.5 standard deviations below the norm after treatment. His efficiency (throughput) on the second administration was average (slightly below the mean) at pretreatment and improved to almost 1.5 standard deviations above average after treatment.

Initial learning improved significantly on Trial 1 of AVLT, from >3 standard deviations below average in the pretreatment phase to +0.5 standard deviations following treatment (Fig. 6.67). Performance was better on three of the five trials following treatment. After a 30 minute delay, recall improved from −0.6 standard

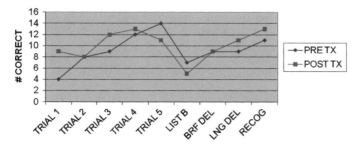

Fig. 6.67 HJ AVLT performance

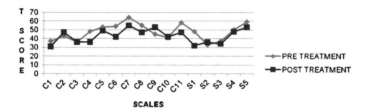

Fig. 6.68 HJ pre versus posttreatment scores on LNNB

deviations before treatment to +1.7 standard deviations following treatment, a gain of 2.3 standard deviations. Recognition improved by two words following treatment (from −3 standard deviations to −1.5 standard deviations). The improvements on these learning and memory tasks suggested that attention was an important contributor to the memory deficits.

On the LNNB lower T scores reflected better performance and a regression equation using age and education determined expected performance on an individual basis. The normal range for HJ was 35–55T. Impairment (S5) improved from mildly impaired to normal, but this change, while it may be clinically significant, represented an improvement of 0.5 standard deviations and was not statistically significant (Fig. 6.68). Intellectual processing (C11) showed a significant improvement from mildly impaired to average ($p < 0.01$).

The neuropsychological profile suggested some scores (attention, accuracy, learning, intellectual processes) had consistently returned to normal while others showed inconsistent improvement. Processing speed was normal on LNNB but slow on PASAT and varied by type of material on Stroop.

Regarding ecological validity, HJ applied to a University and was accepted as a full-time student.

Treatment of Attention

These cases illustrated that attention problems in the postacute phase can be readily improved. This included sustained, alternating, and divided attention.

It was also clear that memory sequelae following head injury may be due to attentional problems (i.e., the encoding stage of memory) and that addressing attention in these two cases was sufficient to restore normal memory functions. Resumption of a normal life following treatment was demonstrated by both cases as well.

Executive Functioning

SJ was a 52-year-old physician who was a rear seat passenger in a vehicle that was struck from behind by a second vehicle traveling at 50 miles per hour while the impacted vehicle was moving at 5 miles per hour. The patient reported whiplash but no loss of consciousness. The following day she had a stiff neck, severe headache, and blurred vision. She nonetheless returned to work and for the next 2 days experienced visual disturbances and perseverative, illogical speech.

Quantitative Electroencephalography 1 month post-injury demonstrated diffuse low voltage activity in all frequency bands. While beta activity may be subject to a muscle artifact, this is not the case for alpha and theta waves. Relative power for all regions was low for alpha and excessive for theta. Theta was especially excessive in all frontal leads. Extreme asymmetry and hypocoherence were found for the frequency bands between the occipital areas and temporal and parietal regions. Anterior regions tended to have more power on the right side. Interhemispheric gradients were disturbed, with statistically significant excessive posterior beta activity. There were small sharp waves in the right parietal and occipital regions. P300 was normal in the anterior regions but completely absent bilaterally from posterior temporal, parietal and occipital regions. The profile suggested a postconcussion syndrome.

Three months post injury she was administered neuropsychological tests, which revealed visual and auditory oversensitivities, generalized memory retrieval problems, mild-to-moderately severe bilateral fine motor dyspraxias, marked tactile-spatial reasoning deficits, conceptual inflexibility and difficulties reasoning in ambiguous, unstructured situations. The neuropsychologist felt the pattern of deficits suggested occipitoparietal and bilateral prefrontal dysfunction. One month later an optometrist concluded that head trauma had interrupted her ability to perceive and manage visual–spatial functions. She spent the next year in treatment with a developmental opthamologist followed by neurofeedback to alter her QEEG. She had been unable to return to practice since the injury. She frequently burned herself while cooking because she was so easily distracted.

At this point she was administered a neuropsychological test battery as a basis for a cognitive remediation treatment plan. Intellectual functioning was in the superior range, processing speed was below average, and conceptual linguistic functioning was mildly impaired. Reasoning and flexibility, sequencing social situations, and sorting (all executive functions) were impaired. Visual spatial reasoning was unimpaired. Attention to detail was low average.

Attention and executive functions were targeted. After about a year of weekly sessions her attorney insisted that she have an interim retesting. The results were as follows. Intellectual functioning improved to "Very Superior", visual spatial reasoning was significantly improved from baseline, attention to details was significantly improved, and sequencing social situations and sorting were markedly improved. Reasoning and flexibility had not been treated yet and her scores were unchanged in this area. She continued treatment until meeting all criteria set for her after which a final testing was repeated (all testings were done by an independent neuropsychologist who had referred her for treatment but had no information about what deficits she had been working on or her level of achievement in treatment at the interim or final testing.) She continued to show improvement on testing.

During the course of treatment she had been told by her doctors to forget about return to work as a physician or a professional of any sort. They recommended work at a convenience store. She was extremely upset and we spoke about the goals we had and that it was entirely too soon to determine the level at which she would eventually be able to function. Her doctors were assuming that there could be no recovery after the acute phase of injury, as this is what they were taught. As time proceeded and she felt she was improving, she arranged to work under the supervision of another physician. She made a diagnosis missed by her supervisor and was doing well under supervision. However, she and her supervisor agreed she was not ready to practice independently. Unfortunately, the supervisor retired and she could find no other physician to set up an individualized program as the last one had done. By the interim testing, she was no longer burning herself when working in the kitchen.

Another case of executive dysfunction was MD, a 30-year-old, self-employed man who purchased, renovated, and resold houses. He also researched patents and was a graduate student who had completed all coursework for his doctorate. He was about to begin work on his dissertation when an 18-wheeler ran him off the road. He lost consciousness briefly, was treated in an ER, and was then released. On two subsequent occasions he returned to the ER because of nausea, vomiting, abdominal pain, headache, and syncope. CT scan was normal, as is usually the case with concussions. Four months post injury he still suffered from headaches, slowed mental processing, difficulties with sustaining attention, and memory problems.

Neuropsychological testing revealed problems in attention, processing speed, abstract thinking, and memory. With regard to attention and processing speed, the Seashore Rhythm scale, Trails A and Trails B all fell below a T of 40. Speech Sound was $T = 45$. Digit Span Scale Score was 10 while Digit Symbol was 8. Reasoning and abstract thinking on the Categories Test produced a T score of 43, far below expectation for this highly educated and intelligent man. Learning and memory were impaired on the CVLT ($T = 17$).

Attempts to remediate attention and processing speed with *Get Q and Two in One* were unsuccessful because he was unable to speed his performance on tasks with numbers and letters as they looked "school-related". He performed the tasks

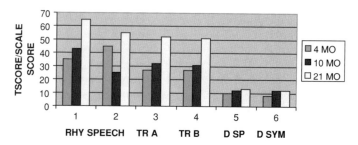

Fig. 6.69 M.D. tests of attention

extremely slowly so that he would be accurate, and he felt anxious speeding up for fear of making mistakes. We therefore used *Space Probe, Dartboard,* and *Run Silent* to help improve attention and processing speed, as they do not resemble academic work. Reasoning exercises included *Detective* and *Mission Decode.* Memory strategies were taught on *Symbol Memory, Line Up, Concentration, Memory Game* 2, and *Shopping List.*

Criteria for normal speed and accuracy were met on all levels of *Space Probe, Dartboard,* and *Run Silent.* He proceeded from a presentation speed (speed at which the rocket travels) of 4 to a speed of 10 on *Space Probe* and increased presentation speed from 10 to 15 on *Dartboard.* He was eventually able to score not only within normal limits but also to throw the darts accurately every time, despite the rapid rate at which they appeared. He also met criteria for the abstract reasoning exercises. He learned to use a verbal strategy on the visual memory exercise *Symbol Memory.* After five sessions he was taught to gradually rely less on the compensatory mechanism and increasingly on visualizing. Performance demonstrated effective use of the compensatory strategy and the eventual restoration of his visual memory, which had been clearly impaired following his injury. All memory exercises were practiced until he reached criteria for normal performance. For example, he learned all lists on *Shopping List* to 100% accuracy using the strategies he was taught.

Retesting demonstrated improved attention/processing (Fig. 6.69). Digit Span improved from a scaled score of 10 to a score of 12 following attention training. A final retesting at the completion of the entire remediation program produced a scaled score of 13 (SS = 13). Digit Symbol improved from a scaled scored of 8 to 12 following attention training. This level of performance was maintained at the end of remediation. Luria Rhythm improved from a T of 35 to 43 following attention training and 65 by the end of remediation (Luria Ts were converted so that higher Ts were better). Speech Sounds was $T = 45$ pretreatment, $T = 25$ following attention training and $T = 55$ on completion of remediation. Trail Making A and B showed a steady improvement from pretreatment to post-attention training to posttreatment when scores exceeded Ts of 50.

No explicit remediation was attempted in the area of sensorimotor functioning. On Grooved Pegboard the dominant hand improved somewhat, from $T = 23$ to 28.

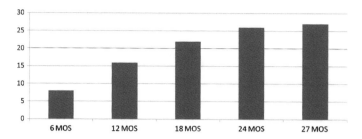

Fig. 6.70 M.D. work performance: average number of patents pulled per hour

Nondominant hand showed a mild decrement following treatment ($T = 36$ versus $T = 32$). Tactile Performance Test with the dominant hand improved from $T = 31$ to 35). The nondominant hand improved from $T = 28$ to 45. Both hands showed mild improvement from $T = 30$ to 35. Nondominant hand performance on TPT seemed to be the only improvement that was likely not due to test–retest variability and all other scores remained clearly impaired.

Reasoning improved on the Category Test from $T = 40$ to 49 at mid point of remediation and $T = 46$ at the end of training, suggesting statistically nonsignificant improvement. Verbal learning and memory on CVLT were not improved by general memory strategies learned on *Symbol Memory*, *Concentration*, and *Line Up* ($T = 25$ at pretraining to $T = 12$ post general memory training).

He was then given training on *Memory Game* 2 and *Shopping List*, which present several list learning strategies. Thereafter, his CVLT score improved to $T = 35$, a full standard deviation above his performance before learning the new strategies. All testing was done by the neuropsychologist who had referred him and at time frames dictated by the patient's attorney, independent of phase of treatment or progress in treatment. The tester did not know what cognitive areas had been completed, except that the final testing was after treatment had been discontinued.

The patient reported significant improvement in his visual memory, to about 80% of his excellent premorbid level. He had kept meticulous work records on the number of patents he was able to pull per hour for his research, dating from pre-injury throughout the course of treatment (Fig. 6.70). Prior to his injury he had averaged 30 patents per hour. Six months post injury he was averaging 12 per hour. About 27 months post injury he was pulling 27 patents per hour, approaching his premorbid functioning. He had written and published a professional paper during the course of treatment and consulted to a movie company on the use of objects authentic to the period that was the subject of the film. He and his wife felt he had made excellent progress through cognitive remediation, although he had not fully returned to premorbid functioning.

Another instance of executive dysfunction was WM who was impulsive and used poor judgment following his head injury. He was a 19-year-old, high-school educated construction worker who fell from a moving truck and was confined to intensive care for 2 weeks. He spent a week-and-a-half on the Brain Injury Unit of a hospital after which he was transferred to a rehabilitation hospital for another 2 weeks. CT Scan revealed right frontoparietal hemorrhagic contusion. There was also left ossicular disruption associated with hearing loss and visual edema. He was placed on Celexa to help manage depression. He reported short-temperedness.

Neuropsychological testing was done 4 months post injury. At the time he had a 24-hour retrograde amnesia and several days anterograde amnesia. Testing revealed impulsive responding, stimulus screening problems, distractibility, need for structure, attention/concentration difficulties, and a left-sided tactile processing problem. However, 1 month later, without further testing, he was discharged as fit for work without restriction. An independent contracter found him fit to drive. He was fired from his job and was in a hit-and-run accident the first time he drove. He reported he did not know he hit the other vehicle.

Seven months post injury he was again administered a neuropsychological testing battery. He was found to have an incomplete recovery from head injury, marked by inconsistency and variability in performance. One story was remembered well but a comparable one was not. He had highly variable scores on interference tasks. For example, Trigrams was at the 4th percentile for a 9-second delay but at the 58th percentile for a 36-second delay. Focused auditory attention was normal on Speech Sounds and Seashore Rhythm. Sustained visual attention on Stroop was impaired for verbal material (2nd percentile) but not for nonverbal material (31st percentile). Judgment was good on the Wisconsin Card Sort (82nd percentile), WAIS III Comprehension (75th percentile), and WAIS III Picture Arrangement (50th percentile).

A NeurXercise program was devised to address concentration, distractibility, and impulsivity. In addition he was assigned a psychotherapist to help him focus on daily problems in these areas and his lack of insight as sources of problems for him. Concentration, distraction, and impulse control are involved in *Get Q* and his baseline on this exercise suggested he might benefit from working on it. Sustained attention (concentration), alternating attention (requires freedom from distraction), and perseveration (a manifestation of impulsive responding and inability to shift set) are practiced on *Two in One*, so this was also included in his treatment plan. *Run Silent* 3 and 4 include the same requirements so these were added as well. *Dartboard* 2 was added for additional practice on sustained attention. Freedom from distraction and ability to divide his attention and multitask was practiced on *Double Trouble*. Cognitive flexibility and resistance to impulsive responding were addressed on *Mission Decode*.

Speed on *Get Q* 2 improved from mildly impaired to normal (see Online Resource 66). Accuracy was quite variable, but by the last two sessions his performance was more consistent and within the normal range, whereas he had begun highly variable and outside of normal limits in the first two sessions, normal the next two sessions, abnormal the next session, and finally within normal limits again during the last two sessions (see Online Resource 67). Since he performed within normal limits during four of the last five sessions, it was felt that he met the criteria for discontinuing the exercise. Whereas consistent normal performance on *Get Q* 2 took seven sessions to reach, speed and accuracy on the more demanding *Get Q* 3 took only three sessions, suggesting transfer of training or generalization

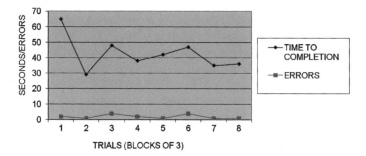

Fig. 6.71 WM sustained and alternating attention: Two in One ¾

(see Online Resources 68 and 69). *Two in One* 1 criterion was met in seven trials (two at baseline and the rest the following week). Speed and accuracy on this attention and impulse control task are depicted in Online Resource 70. *Two in One* 2 was completed in the same number of sessions but with twice as many trials (see Online Resource 71). On *Two in One* 3 Fig. 6.71 shows his baseline trial under trial 1 and blocks of three trials constitute the other data points. After seven blocks of three trials (i.e., 21 trials total) his performance was consistently within the expected range. He practiced *Run Silent* 3 for seven trials, the last four of which met the criterion for successful attention and impulse control. He was then given the highly demanding *Run Silent* 4, which randomly changes the height of the plane and the depth of the submarine on each run within a trial. His performance was highly variable and far from meeting the criterion for success (see Online Resource 72).

He then missed 2 weeks of treatment and did not practice during that time. He was readministered *Run Silent* 3 to ensure that he had not lost ground. Online Resource 73 shows that he performed poorly and never duplicated his previous level of performance (only trial 13 of the 14 trials was comparable to his per-formance of 2 weeks earlier.) Online Resource 74 shows sustained attention performance on *Dartboard* 2. He was highly variable in his performance and did not reach the criterion of two consecutive performances averaging more than 90 points until trial 23. Despite the decrement in his performance, he felt he was doing well. He dropped out of treatment, left his parent's home to live in his girlfriend's parents' house and sought new employment as he had been fired from his recent job because he left without informing anyone. He failed to get another job and stress built at his girlfriend's house. After 6 months he negotiated with his parents for return to their home under the stipulation that he return to treatment and follow house rules.

His performance on *Run Silent* 3 was initially at the reduced level seen after his 2 week hiatus. However, he was able to return to the criterion level, as he had earlier in the treatment program (see Fig. 6.72). *Get Q* 2 and 3 were at the normal levels seen 6 months earlier. Similarly, *Two in One* 1, 2, 3, and 4 were performed within normal limits after 6 months without intervening practice. Thus,

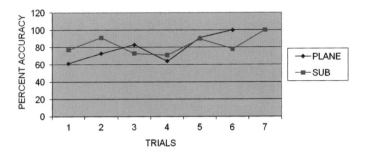

Fig. 6.72 WM alternating attention/visual motor tracking: Run Silent 3 (after 6 months of not practicing)

performance on many of the exercises had not shown a deterioration over 6 months. The one exercise that deteriorated after 2 weeks without practice remained deteriorated after 6 months but returned to normal levels after only seven practice trials (three 1 week and four the next).

We next undertook problem solving and cognitive flexibility as reflected in the ability to generate and test hypotheses and to shift set when feedback so indicated. *Mission Decode* 1 was practiced for eight sessions (see Online Resource 75). Six of the eight sessions met the criterion of fewer than six errors (0–3 misses on trials 3–8). A more complex version of the same task, utilizing more difficult principles, was next undertaken. *Mission Decode* 2 was also completed in eight trials. He struggled with this more difficult exercise but reached the criterion of fewer than six errors by the eighth trial (see Online Resource 76). Generalization was seen in his taking the same amount of time to pass a more difficult exercise with more complex principles.

Multitasking on *Double Trouble* 2 was practiced to a goal of 800 points (see Online Resource 77). The criterion was to average over 89 points per rocket launch while making no errors on the tonal discrimination task. He met the criterion on trials 3 and 4, and 6 and 7. The number of points, and therefore time spent multitasking, was increased to 1,000. He reached the criterion by trial 2 (see Online Resource 78). The goal was then increased to 2,000 points. Online Resource 79 demonstrates that he met the criterion on four of the five trials practiced. He was told to practice the exercise to 5,000 points and if he succeeded to increase the goal to 10,000 points. He agreed to do so. He left for his psychotherapy appointment and returned in about an hour to do his assignment. He practiced one trial at 2,000 points, two trials at 3,000 points and ran *Mission Decode*, which he had completed during our session and was not part of his assignment. After about 15 minutes of unobserved practice in which he did none of the assigned tasks, he left for the day.

Over the course of the next two sessions his performance on *Double Trouble* 2 was variable with regard to accuracy of responding to the notes, but he consistently met the criterion for 5,000 points by session 3 (see Online Resource 80) in which points increased to an average of 93 while missed notes dropped to an average of

0.6 during the third session). On this last session his score never dropped below 90 and four of seven trials were errorless. He then practiced the same task to 10,000 points, about 10 minutes of sustained and divided attention. He met the criterion on the very first trial. He then switched to *Double Trouble* 1 set to 10,000 points and easily met the criterion for success, reflecting skill transfer and generalization. Thereafter, he attended four more sessions working unsuccessfully on *Run Silent* 4. He then began to miss sessions so a retesting was scheduled.

Performance was no longer variable on Trigrams and PASAT. Sustained attention improved. Performance on the 1990s version of ANAM improved by more than a standard deviation, returning to the normal range. Sustained attention to verbal material on Stroop improved from 31st percentile to the 53rd. With nonverbal material Stroop improved from the 2nd percentile to the 18th. Auditory processing on PASAT improved from the 24th to the 50th percentile. Divided attention on Trigrams improved at the 9-second delay (4th percentile to 81st percentile) and 18-second delay (31st to 72nd percentile). There was no change at the 36-second delay (58th percentile). Executive functioning also improved dramatically. Emotional responding was no longer present during testing on LNNB and PASAT. Perseverations were no longer excessive on Trigrams and AVLT. Set shifting was within normal limits on PASAT. Resistance to distraction on AVLT (short delay condition) improved from the 69th percentile to the 96th percentile). Reduced impulsivity and better judgment were seen in his performing more slowly but more accurately.

A real-life reflection of improved impulse control and judgment occurred when a snowstorm was forecast for the day he was scheduled for posttreatment testing. He telephoned a few days in advance and asked if he could reschedule the testing if the roads were bad on the appointment date. This reflected forethought and appreciation of the importance of the testing. The storm was much milder than predicted and he arrived on time without having to reschedule. He had been working for his father, at first traveling with him when he did not have his own transportation and thereafter on his own when he had saved enough money to purchase his own vehicle. No accidents or problems while driving were reported. He was trying to save money in anticipation of marrying his girlfriend.

Treatment of Executive Dysfunction

The case of SJ, like that of CG discussed under *Subcortical disorders*, suggests that NeurXercise and other treatments may potentiate and speed up the positive effects seen with each treatment separately. Reasoning was clearly improved, as exemplified by her ability to deduce a diagnosis that was missed by her supervisor and other physicians. MD improved his ability to plan, organize, and execute, as seen in his ability to write and publish a paper, consult to a movie company, and to research and pull appropriate patents in an accurate and speedy fashion. WM demonstrated many problems with impulsivity and judgment, but after his cognitive remediation was completed and he was scheduled for retesting, he behaved

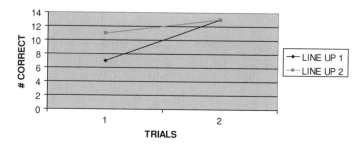

Fig. 6.73 LM facial memory: Lineup

in an appropriate and non-impulsive manner. Thus, these cases of executive dysfunction reflected real-life improvement in reasoning, judgment, and impulse control.

Memory

LM was a 27-year-old left-handed college educated woman who worked in government contracting when she was in an automobile accident. She was hit on the driver's side and forced off the road where she hit a speed limit sign and telephone pole. She lost consciousness between the time she hit the pole and her removal from the wreck by emergency medical technicians. She sustained ligament damage, knee, and hip injuries and required 60 stitches to her open head injury. Two months later she had a blowout on the road, safely got to the shoulder, and then had a panic attack. She was evaluated with a neuropsychological testing battery beginning 3 months post-injury and testing was completed 4 months post injury. It was determined that she was suffering from PTSD as well as incomplete recovery from her head injury. It was recommended that she be referred for cognitive remediation after the PTSD had successfully resolved.

Three months later (7 months post-injury) she was referred for cognitive remediation by her psychiatrist who felt the PTSD was no longer an issue.

Her neuropsychological testing results revealed diffuse bilateral dysfunction, mild impairment, and incomplete compensation. Processing speed was slow but accurate. Immediate verbal memory was severely impaired, but there was significant variability in list learning, story memory, and visual nonverbal memory. Delayed memory approached average on list learning and visual reproduction. After attention was remediated, memory was targeted. She was administered *Line Up* 2 and 3 for facial memory, *Concentration* for object memory, and *Shopping List* for list memory.

She learned the strategies taught on *Shopping List* very quickly. However, she had more difficulty with nonverbal memory. Facial memory strategies and practice were the focus on *Line Up*. Figure 6.73 demonstrates that she made a dramatic

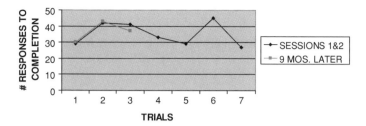

Fig. 6.74 LM visual memory for objects: Concentration 1

improvement in identification of the photograph to which she had been exposed (*Line Up* 1), correctly identifying almost twice as many as she had at baseline. When she had to keep in mind all the photographs flashed and identify which of the choices were not among them (*Line Up* 2), improvement was slight. Recalling the locations of objects is the goal in *Concentration* 1. Figure 6.74 shows performance at baseline (trials 1–5), the following week (trials 6–7), and 9 months thereafter (the second graph, containing three trials). Of her ten practice trials, only three approached the normal range of no more than 20–28 trials needed to match the objects (trial 1, trial 7, and the first trial after 9 months had elapsed.)

Repeat neuropsychological testing demonstrated improvement in verbal memory but worsening of or no change in nonverbal memory, consistent with her NeurXercise performance. List learning on AVLT improved on the final learning trial (Trial 5) from 11 words to 14 out of 15 words recalled, and following the distracter list (Immediate Recall) from 7 words to 11 of 15 words recalled. Recognition after a 30-minute delay was perfect. However, the recognition trial was not administered initially so no comparison can be made to determine whether this represented an improvement over baseline. List learning on LNNB also improved. She made ten errors on the initial testing (impaired performance) and six at posttreatment (borderline normal). Story memory improved as well. On the LNNB story she initially recalled only two bits of information (impaired performance). Posttreatment recall was seven bits of information (normal performance). Her pretreatment WMS-R immediate recall was below average (16th percentile) but WMS III posttreatment performance for immediate story recall was average (44th percentile). After a 30 minute delay WMS III was better than baseline WMS-R, although both were below normal (3rd versus 15th percentile). WMS-R Visual Reproduction I, taken at baseline, was above average (90% correct). The WMS III version of this test, which is more difficult, was performed at the impaired range (64% correct). There was a slight improvement from WMS-R delayed memory to WMS III delayed recall. The difference between these two versions of the test were great, as can be seen by the fact that she scored in a higher percentile on WMS III delayed memory with 37% correct than on WMS-R with 66% correct. It seems inadvisable to try to compare these two tests.

The patient reported that the remediation program had taught her compensatory skills that served her on the job. She was most concerned about losing her job because of her memory problems when she entered treatment. Following treatment she reported that the strategies helped and that she was performing her duties successfully. She reported that she had the treatment to thank for keeping her job.

Treatment of Memory Deficits

This case illustrated that at least some memory problems can be successfully remediated through the development of compensatory skills following a serious open head wound, even after the acute phase of recovery. Other instances of successful remediation of memory were cited earlier. For example, the case of AF (under *Head trauma*) demonstrated significant improvement following training in compensatory memory strategies. The case of MD (under *Executive functioning*) reflects the successful application of remediation techniques for restitution of memory functions that had been impaired by closed head injury.

Short-term memory deficits are the most common memory complaints and cognitive remediation has been successful in improving short-term retention with verbal, visual, and spatial materials. Benefits have been shown to last after delays of 30 minutes on many standardized tests and up to 3 hours or more on the LNNB. Patients report improvement in daily short-term memory.

Subpopulations

Obviously, there are other ways to look at the populations we assess and treat other than etiology and cognitive domains. The results of cognitive remediation remain consistent across subpopulations as well. For example, older patients have been found to respond well to cognitive remediation, e.g., KP under *Co-morbid conditions* and the cases cited below.

Geriatrics

A 57-year-old psychiatrist suffered a mild closed head injury and was treated for sustained attention problems. Prior to treatment he complained that he could only concentrate for a few minutes on his journals while at posttreatment he complained he could only concentrate for an hour or two (!). He had a life-long problem remembering names and faces, which was substantiated at baseline when he could recall only 2 or 3 out of 10 name-face pairs over four different groupings (9 out of 40 remembered). Following training in the peg-word system on *What's My Name*, he was able to get 100% correct or 40 out of 40.

A 67-year-old retired phone company technician had cognitive deficits secondary to cerebrovascular disease. Processing speed was practiced on *Get Q* 1, 2, and 3 and *Two in One* 1 and 2, all of which were impaired at baseline testing. He was taught a self-cuing strategy that led to normal processing on *Get Q* 1 in just two sessions. He did equally well on Level 2 after two sessions. Generalization was seen when he mastered the more difficult processing task on Level 3 in just one session and was able to bring his performance up to normal levels on *Two in One* 1 and 2 within a single session. Impaired spatial ability was addressed successfully with NeurXercise and he did well on increasingly difficult tasks. Memory for faces on *Line Up* 1 improved to normal in just one session. Level 2 reached normal after three sessions. Spatial memory on *Concentration* improved about 50% when he became ill and had to discontinue treatment.

A 67-year-old elementary school principal had to retire after breaking his arm and sustaining a head injury while playing tennis. A few months later he began to experience headaches at the site of the impact and noticed his memory was failing. Testing done 13 months post-accident revealed impairment localized to the site of the head injury. Six months thereafter he was tested again and a decline in functioning was noted in processing speed, visual–spatial organization, visual memory and intellectual functioning. After 5 weeks there was noticeable improvement in processing speed on *Get Q* 1 and one of the trials during the fifth session was actually within normal limits. A few weeks thereafter speed and accuracy were within normal limits. *Get Q* 2 was practiced using a verbal cuing strategy and he met the criterion after six sessions. He mastered *Get Q* 3 after only three sessions. *Two in One* was within normal speed and accuracy after five sessions for Level 1 and after four sessions for Level 2. *Get Q* has a visual–spatial element that is practiced in addition to processing speed. His wife reported that following the above training his driving had improved and that he did not drive so close to the lines demarcating the lanes. He labored for some time on a visual/spatial-executive function task before mastering it. Thereafter, he mastered comparable tasks within a few sessions, suggesting generalization of the skill. Memory for strings of words on *Memory Game* 2 improved from inconsistently recalling up to four words to 93% accuracy on strings of six words. *Line Up* 1 was 10 of 18 faces recalled at baseline and 12 of 18 following list learning on *Memory Game* 2. One session of facial recall training led to 16 of 18 recalled. Thus, he improved on tasks measuring processing speed, executive functioning, visual–spatial organization, and memory.

Attention Deficit Disorder

BX was a 26-year-old who was diagnosed with ADHD at age six or seven and was on Ritalin until the sixth grade. He reported daydreaming and having difficulty studying in high school. He was working full time and taking college classes but last year he found himself bored and staring off in class. This year he changed jobs.

The new job was much more demanding and required significantly more multi-tasking. He found himself behind and having to rush to get everything done by the end of the day. He was also finding his college courses difficult. He had been married for 3 years. He had some family-related stresses but these were resolved. His school and work problems, however, did not resolve.

Neuropsychological testing included WAIS III subtests (Working Memory Index), Wechsler Memory Scale III (Logical Memory I and II), Conners' CPT, Wisconsin Card Sorting Test, AVLT, Stroop, Auditory Consonant Trigrams, PASAT, Trail Making Test, and Controlled Oral Word Association. He was found to be impulsive on Conners' CPT. His AVLT demonstrated slow learning and retroactive interference.

WAIS III Working Memory Index was in the superior range as were all three subtests that made it up (Arithmetic, Digit Span, and Letter Number Sequencing).

PASAT scores were above average to superior. Visual attention on Trails A was above average. Stroop was average for visual attention and executive functioning.

Multitasking on Trigrams was above average to superior. Wisconsin Card Sort scores were within normal limits and freedom from perseveration was superior. Set shifting on Trails B was superior. Controlled Oral Word Association was average for generating words beginning with designated letters but below average for words belonging to a designated category. Story memory was average for immediate and delayed conditions.

The treatment plan addressed impulsivity, learning speed, and executive functions (e.g., problem solving, rapid set shifting, rapid processing, and multi-tasking with two and three tasks performed simultaneously for longer periods of time). Impulse control was practiced on *Two in One* Levels 3. Problem solving and learning were practiced on *Detective, Mission Decode*, and *Tower of Hanoi*. Set shifting exercises included *Two in One* 3 and 4, *Run Silent* 3, *Detective* and *Mission Decode*. Processing speed was involved in *Dartboard* and *Double Trouble*. Visual/spatial memory and learning were practiced on *Concentration*.

Following baselines, he was able to produce a flawless performance within a normal speed on *Two in One 3*. He solved the Tower of Hanoi problem in four attempts following baseline, producing the ideal solution on trial 4. During the treatment phase he took only two trials to get a perfect score on *Mission Decode* 1 and he was within normal limits after two trials on Level 2. That is, he did not blow up on trials 3 or 4 during which the number of errors was under five. His score was within normal limits on the initial trials following baseline, performed a month after the abnormal baseline was obtained. Improved set shifting ability was seen on the above performances on *Two in One, Detective* and *Mission Decode*. He was able to meet criterion on *Run Silent* 3 after only three trials during the treatment phase. The processing speed criterion was quickly met on *Dartboard*. Levels 1 and 2 of *Double Trouble* were easily performed to criterion. When a third task was introduced for simultaneous processing, his excellent scores did not change. While visual–spatial memory was below criterion at baseline, he easily met the criterion during treatment.

He began treatment with the spatial problem, *Tower of Hanoi*. After meeting the criterion he quickly dispensed with the mental–spatial, impulse control task, *Two in One* 3. Practice with these spatial tasks seems to have generalized as he quickly mastered *Run Silent* 3. This further seemed to have generalized to visual processing as he took only two trials to master *Dartboard*. Multitasking was a complaint he had had, but his testing did not support this as a problem area. He demonstrated superior performance on two and three task exercises. Visual set shifting on *Run Silent* 3 and problem solving on *Tower of Hanoi* seem to have generalized to the problem solving, set shifting tasks of *Detective* and *Mission Decode*, the last exercises to be practiced.

Retesting was limited to the CPT, Stroop, AVLT, and Controlled Oral Word Association, as he had done so well at baseline on the other measures. The following changes occurred. There was no longer any indicator of impulsivity on CPT. His Stroop interference score, which measures impulse control, improved from average (75th percentile) to superior (93rd percentile). Retroactive interference on AVLT was no longer present (his score went from the 20th percentile to the 80th percentile on List A Short Delay). There was no change in word generation on Controlled Oral Word Association, which was not addressed in the treatment plan, suggesting that the other changes were due to the intervention and not across the board improvement due to practice effects on the tests.

At the conclusion of treatment BX reported that he was having no trouble completing his work on time. He felt he was a little distracted when he began in the morning but that this quickly disappeared and he worked efficiently and effectively through the day. Prior to treatment he had reported that he was distracted for about the first half of the day and then had to work feverishly to get done.

Symptoms and Mechanisms in Attention Deficit (Hyperactivity) Disorder

The American Psychiatric Association (2000) identifies ADHD as characterized by symptoms of hyperactivity, impulsivity, and inattention. Estimates of the continuance into adulthood have ranged from 4 to 75%, with a recent study (Barkley et al. 2002) concluding that persistence into adulthood has been underestimated. Studies suggest that up to 50% of children with a parent diagnosed with ADHD display the symptoms. There is no research that examines the psychological effects of being raised by an ADHD parent on producing ADHD-like behaviors as opposed to the assumption that it must be genetic. Hervey et al. (2004) did a meta-analysis of adult ADHD research and identified the neuropsychological tests that best discriminated adults with ADHD from control groups. These tests were drawn from the domains of response inhibition, memory, executive functioning, processing and motor speed, and intelligence. The tests used in the above case of BX drew upon the results of that research. Possible mechanisms of ADHD include neurotransmitter systems (norepinephrine and dopamine have been implicated), reticular activating system-frontal lobe localization (Luria's Principle Functional Unit 1), neural circuitry (frontostriatal and frontocerebellar) or non-neurological etiology. Premotor and superior prefrontal cortices have been implicated in PET studies examining adults who have been hyperactive since childhood. The evidence is building that ADHD is a neurological disorder. However, mechanisms are unknown although there are many, wide-ranging possibilities. It is important to note that, like other neurological disorders, it can be effectively treated with cognitive remediation and medication may not be necessary.

BX initially presented with impulse control issues that were greater than expected in light of his general above average to superior cognitive abilities. Executive dysfunction was seen in problems with set shifting and problem solving. He did not display the working memory difficulties that are often seen. His sustained attention problems were minor and seen mostly on CPT.

Learning Disability

KR was a 22-year-old woman with documented reading problems and a history of placement in a learning disabilities class in high school. Her scores were "low" on SAT. She completed college as a Biology major with a 3.3 average. However, she could not get better than a C in History or English. She had taken the MCAT exam on several occasions but was never able to complete more than 7 of 10 passages and had trouble answering questions on the passages she completed due to impaired comprehension when she tried to read quickly.

Medical history was positive for being hit on the head with a hammer by her sister when she was a child. She reported there was a visible bump and she was treated at a hospital. While in high school she was in an MVA and hit her head on the windshield. She reported redness around the right eye as the only symptom at that time.

Baseline neuropsychological testing showed mild to moderate impairment on the LNNB with excellent compensation. Processing speed and overall accuracy were mildly impaired. Intellectual functioning was low average due to difficulties attending to details, slow processing speed, and variability on verbal abstract reasoning tasks.

Immediate memory for verbal material was mildly impaired on LNNB while immediate visual–nonverbal memory was within normal limits. Delayed memory after 3-hours was variable. Attention to audioverbal material was impaired while nonverbal material was attended to well. Word generation was below the 5th percentile on FAS. Reading was slow with occasional errors.

The treatment plan addressed attention to detail, verbal memory, and executive functioning. To improve attention to verbal material she worked on *Get Q* 1 and *Two in One* Levels 1, 2, and 3. Verbal memory strategies, including "chunking", visual coding, and creating a story containing key words to be recalled, were

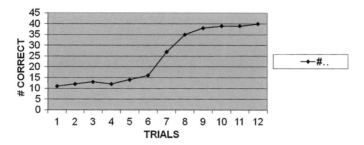

Fig. 6.75 KR verbal and nonverbal reasoning: Mission Decode 2

taught and practiced on *Memory Game* 2 and *Shopping List*. Executive functions targeted were verbal and nonverbal reasoning and verbal and nonverbal judgment.

Online Resource 81 demonstrates that focused attention was at the mean for the normative group on the first two trials and improved from there on 6 of the next seven trials. She showed significant improvement over baseline on all levels of *Two in One* (see Online Resources 82–84). Performance speed improved far beyond normative levels and was more accurate.

List learning strategies were taught on *Memory Game* 2 while study time for the lists was extended. Online Resource 85 shows that there was improvement on the first session, greater improvement during the second session, and near perfect performance by the third session. For the final session the speed of presentation or time allotted for study was increased to the level used when collecting normative data. She demonstrated perfect performance for both presentations of the list. She then practiced *Shopping List* (see Online Resource 86). It took four trials to master the first list, two trials to master the second, four to master the third, and only one to master the fourth list.

Online Resource 87 depicts verbal reasoning on *Detective* 2 (verbal analogies). She began making three errors on the first two trials, one error on trial 3, and no errors on the next two trials. Online Resource 88 demonstrates performance on pictorial problem solving as practiced on *Mission Decode* Level 1. Baseline performance was poor while there was a substantial improvement on the next trial. Thereafter, she completed the program without detonating the bomb. The last three trials were performed without error. On *Mission Decode* Level 2 both nonverbal and verbal problem solving were incorporated. She demonstrated an almost classic learning curve, reaching perfect performance by trial 12 (Fig. 6.75).

Nonverbal judgment based upon feedback received on *Golf* Level 2 is seen in Fig. 6.76. By the sixth round of 18 holes she had shot par or below par on 15 of the holes. Both verbal judgment and verbal reasoning were practiced on *Vocabulary* Level 3. She was able to identify 90% of the target words on the third session, 100% by the fourth session, and dropped to 95% accuracy on the fifth session. At this point she was retested.

Impairment on LNNB had improved to the normal range. Processing speed and overall accuracy had also improved to the normal range. She improved on mental

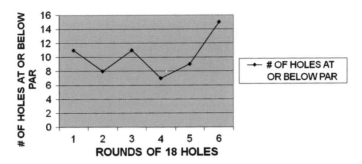

Fig. 6.76 KR judgment: Golf 2

multi-step arithmetic problems. She remained variable on many of the Intellectual Processes items. Immediate verbal memory improved to within normal limits. Performance on story recall and word-picture associations improved but still remained in the impaired range. Delayed memory after 3-hours was now in the normal range. Auditory attention to verbal material improved to normal. Word generation on FAS improved to the normal range (38th percentile). Reading remained unchanged. Thus, major improvement was seen in overall functioning, processing speed, memory, verbal attention and word generation. Executive functions like working memory (multistep mental arithmetic), pictorial sequencing and problem solving, and part–whole relationships showed improvement on LNNB.

Based on these findings it was recommended that she be granted extra time when taking the MCAT. She felt ready to take a speed reading course now that she could attend and process well enough. She did this a few weeks after completing the posttreatment testing and benefited from this training. She was granted time allowances to take the MCAT after my reports were reviewed and did well enough to enter a school of Osteopathy. She required extra time to take her second-year Board exams and this was granted based upon the information I was able to provide.

Another case of learning disability was a 16-year-old girl, EB, who had been home-schooled her whole life. Mother's pregnancy was normal but delivery was protracted over two-and-a-half days. Developmental milestones were all achieved normally. She was described as well-behaved but stubborn. As a younger child she was "quite active". She had trouble sustaining attention, following directions, and expressing herself. She was described as disorganized and having trouble completing tasks. Sense of time and judgment were also problems. She frequently got into physical fights with her sibs and father. She had a long-standing sleep disturbance, marked by initial or terminal insomnia.

Medical history was unremarkable for neurological problems, including head trauma or infection. She had a history of ear infections, beginning in the past 2 years. There were no somatic or visual complaints. She had never been on psychoactive medication. Her family history was positive for speech difficulties on both sides of the family, learning disability in all siblings, and emotional/

behavioral problems. One of her grandparents committed suicide. EB had a history of becoming tearful when expected to readily develop mathematical skills, which were very difficult for her. She reported no concomitant sadness nor any other symptoms suggestive of depression.

Neuropsychological testing revealed normal intelligence in a person with moderate to marked processing deficits and arithmetic learning disability. She had moderately severe deficits on mental numerical reasoning while verbal reasoning skills were average. Performance IQ, dependent on speed of both processing and visual-motor performance, was significantly impaired (standard scores were more than one standard deviation below average for four of the five subtests and Performance IQ was 69). Results of IQ testing suggested nonverbal reasoning deficits and problems reasoning in unstructured situations. Achievement testing on the Wechsler Individual Achievement Test was average for Reading (Standard Score = 102), impaired for Numerical Operations (SS = 63) and below average for Spelling and Written Expression (SS = 80 and 84, respectively).

Sensorimotor testing revealed right fine motor slowing on Finger Tapping and bilateral fine motor dyspraxia and dysgraphia on Purdue Pegboard, drawings, handwriting sample, and Tactile Form Recognition (from the Halstead-Reitan battery). Visual perception was intact on the Stanford-Binet copying task, but visual–spatial orientation was defective on Hooper Visual Organization Test and Benton Judgment of Line Orientation. Auditory discrimination was below expectation for the right ear on the Dichotic Word Listening Test but receptive language processing was unimpaired. Word generation was a problem on Controlled Oral Word Association (FAS) but other expressive language skills were within normal limits (e.g., word definition on Vocabulary subtest, categorical naming on FAS, use of complex language, and confrontational naming on Boston Naming Test).

Sustained attention was significantly impaired on Continuous Performance Task (Vigil K and AK). She was impulsive and slow on the unprimed task but not so under priming conditions. Visual selective attention was variable (deficient to average) and auditory attention to digit and letter spans was below average. Memory testing revealed encoding problems as evidenced by flattened learning curves on Wide Range Assessment of Memory and Learning. She was able to consolidate new visual and auditory information into long-term storage once she had encoded it.

Her psychological profile demonstrated a high degree of defensiveness, resentment, and impulsivity on MMPI-A and Rorschach. Further, the Rorschach suggested problems in the areas of depression and suicide potential. She was referred to a psychiatrist for treatment of depression and to cognitive remediation for the attention, processing, spatial organization, learning/memory, reasoning, and mathematics problems. She refused medication but "talked" regularly with her psychiatrist.

Cognitive remediation began with attention/processing speed training. Focused visual attention on *Get Q* 1 was within the limits suggested in the NeurXercise manual (below 0.6 seconds for reaction time with no more than one error). Her score was better than three of the 14 people in our normal subset. The median score for that

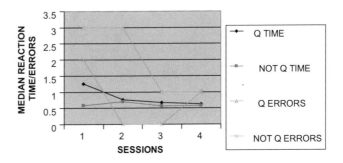

Fig. 6.77   EB alternating and sustained attention: Get Q 2

group was 0.49 seconds and her score was 0.58 seconds. Alternating and sustained visual attention was practiced on *Get Q* Level 2 (see Fig. 6.77). Her baseline performance (plotted as session 1) was slow and inaccurate for both Qs and non-Qs. After three training sessions her score approached normal. Reaction time to Q was equal to or better than three of the 14 normals, was in the recommended range based on normative data (0.5–0.06 seconds) and approached the manual's recommendation of below 0.6 seconds. Reaction time to non-Qs yielded a similar result. Three people from the normative group reacted more slowly and she met the speed recommended in the manual. Errors were reduced to a median of one by the last session. Sustained attention on a visual task, *Dartboard* Level 2, was practiced by having her concentrate on the center of the board and "throw the dart when it reached this point". Online Resource 89 shows that she improved from an average score of 69 points at baseline to an average of 82 points per throw by the last trial of session 2. *Run Silent* Level 3 is an alternating/sustained attention visual–spatial task. Her baseline score was poor so she was trained on each trajectory separately and then returned to the alternating attention task. Online Resource 90 shows that she was able to perform within the recommended guidelines during the second and third sessions (trials 5–6 and trial 7, respectively). Her post baseline scores were significantly better than our normal sample's when they were first exposed to the task, although her baseline scores were significantly worse than normal when she was first exposed to the task (see her baseline score, which is trial 1 on the graph). Prior alternating and sustained attention training seemed to have accelerated her improved performance on this task, suggesting generalization of skills that had initially been impaired.

Learning and encoding were practiced on *Concentration*. Figure 6.78 demonstrates that she met the manual's criterion of matching objects in less than 30 attempts on trials 3–6, after only two substandard performances. The scores on trials 3–6 (location of stimuli are randomly rearranged on each trial) were within a standard deviation of the mean obtained by the normative group (trial 5 was one standard deviation above the norm, trial 4 was at the 50th percentile). *Concentration 2* is the identical task using faces. Generalization of encoding and learning from *Concentration* 1 to 2 can be seen as both trials on Level 2 were within the normal range (trial 1 was a half standard deviation below the mean and trial 2 was

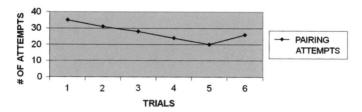

Fig. 6.78 EB visual memory: Concentration 1

a half standard deviation above the mean). Further generalization is suggested by her *Symbol Memory* performance on which she had to recall a sequence of six symbols. She recalled 95%, whereas the normative group had a mean of 84% and standard deviation of 4%. None of the normative group did as well as she did.

Reasoning and problem solving in unstructured situations was addressed with *Mission Decode*, *Detective*, and *Number Guesser* 2. The last exercise involves the use of numbers, which was problematical for her on testing. She was able to solve the unstructured reasoning problems of *Mission Decode* 1 and 2 in four and seven attempts, respectively (see Online Resources 91 and 92). Her final performance was 63 out of 64 and 37 out of 40, respectively. The similarities problems on *Detective* were solved in two attempts, 17 out of 20 and 21 out of 24 (see Online Resource 93). This suggested significant generalization in the use of problem solving strategies in unstructured situations in which the rules changed without notice. On *Number Guesser* 2 she solved the randomly generated number problems in a median of eight trials whereas the normative group did it with a median of seven trials. All scores were within the range produced by a normative group of five college graduates. By the seventh trial she was at the same level as the norm (see Online Resource 94).

She did not undergo posttreatment testing. She was too far behind to pass her grade by the time cognitive remediation was completed. However, she acquitted herself well thereafter, graduated high school, and even went to college. In her first semester she was passing all courses but was slow and behind in submitting her work. The school was working with her when her father lost his job and the family required her to come home as they could no longer afford her college tuition. They were unaware that she had coursework to complete or she would get no credit and she was angry and did not explain the situation well. She got credit for only one course. Approximately 7 years thereafter she again began to take college courses, this time from an online University.

Learning Disability Symptoms and Mechanisms

These cases suggest that people with learning disability may often have underlying problems in attention, processing, and memory. Addressing these issues through cognitive remediation seems to help these individuals function at a significantly higher and more effective level. Intervention produced better reading comprehension and improved reading speed (though not necessarily as fast as their peers). Germano and Capellini (2008) used a program that resulted in their dyslexic patients improving to the level of good readers.

Litigation

In a litigation case following an automobile accident, a 35-year-old woman was stopped at a traffic light when another car hit her and propelled her across a major thoroughfare. She heard her neck snap, feared it might be broken and when she could not get out of the car, she was afraid it would blow up and she would die. She was found to have PTSD and attention and memory problems on evaluation. The Malingering formula on the LNNB suggested that she was not malingering her cognitive symptoms. She was able to improve sustained and alternating attention back into the normal range on *Get Q* and *Two in One* but could not maintain the performance if required to continue on longer lasting tasks. Immediate and short-term memory was practiced until she reached normal functioning. Divided attention training was attempted with *Double Trouble*, but she was never able to successfully perform both tasks simultaneously. She took a job at a much lower level of functioning than she had been used to in order to help pay medical bills and have health insurance while she was waiting for her case to be tried. She was upset that she had such a difficult time with the "simple" clerical tasks involved in her job. She eventually lost the job. Soon thereafter, she was diagnosed with cancer and underwent surgery and chemotherapy. Unfortunately, the attorney she had hired paid little attention to the neurological and psychological aspects of her case, and she did not get compensated for these injuries. The facts that testing found no support for malingering and her attorney was unaware of her involvement in treatment for head injury and PTSD until very shortly before the trial suggested that her prolonged work on cognitive remediation and amelioration of PTSD symptoms was sincere. Unfortunately, the gains were modest and psychological issues kept regressing her to a hopeless, helpless feeling despite cognitive and behavioral gains over the course of treatment.

Another suit involved a 50-year-old woman who sustained brain damage secondary to anoxia suffered during surgery for a hysterectomy. Following surgery, she was treated successfully for depression but her attention and memory problems were unchanged. Two years post surgery CT was normal but evoked potential (P300) was abnormal. Four years post surgery neuropsychological testing revealed attention and memory problems with all other cognitive domains within normal limits. She felt helpless, anxious, and overwhelmed by her report and this was substantiated on the Rorschach. She continued treatment with antidepressants and anxiolytics. Muscle relaxation techniques for the anxiety and NeurXercise for the attention and memory problems were added. She practiced *Two in One* 1 over three sessions, Level 2 over four sessions and Level 3 over two sessions. *Get Q* 1 was mastered in a single session. *Get Q* 2 was practiced for two sessions and Level 3 was worked on for three sessions. *Run Silent* Level 3 was poor at baseline so practice began after she had completed training on Levels 1 and 2. Memory training took place with *Concentration, Line Up* 2 and 3, *Memory Game* 2, and *Shopping List*. Prior to completing the training she moved out of state and discontinued treatment. About 3 years later she contacted me requesting that a copy of her records be forwarded to her attorney. She felt she had made progress with the treatment but that recovery was incomplete.

Chapter 7
Conclusions

The casebook demonstrates that etiology of cognitive symptoms is not the key factor in their remediation. Rather, stability of the neurological condition and availability of alternate functional systems or neural networks are necessary for the intervention to be effective. The number of sessions needed to improve in any identified domain will vary by patient, and the target should be a behavioral and not a temporal one. Following this approach, the casebook demonstrates significant improvement in various kinds of attention and memory problems, visual/spatial deficits, and executive dysfunction, independent of etiology or age of the patient.

Severity and chronicity of injury do not have a negative impact on the likelihood of success with cognitive remediation. As long as there are relatively intact functional systems that can be identified on neuropsychological testing, compensatory and perhaps even restitutional strategies can be successfully implemented. The more chronic the injury, the more likely that emotional factors will be exacerbating the effects of the cognitive impairment. Therefore, one must always consider whether psychotherapy should be part of the treatment plan. Depression, irritability, and anxiety are frequently reported following brain injury and these tend to persist when there has been an incomplete recovery. Headaches are also common sequelae and must be addressed (i.e., medication, biofeedback) if the patient is to be capable of putting forth the necessary effort for recovery.

Finally, neuropsychological testing measures may be insufficient to evaluate true changes in cognitive functioning. There were several cases in which executive functions did not seem to improve following training that targeted these skills, but the patients showed real-life improvements in executive performance. Attention, memory, and visual-spatial tests seem to more frequently show significant changes following cognitive remediation. The casebook reflects that real-life changes are readily documented in these areas following intervention. The changes are seen at work, school, and home.

The casebook provides application of the approach set forth in the first section of the book. This hopefully helps the reader to see how to implement and evaluate

M. H. Podd, *Cognitive Remediation for Brain Injury and Neurological Illness*, 123
DOI: 10.1007/978-1-4614-1975-4_7, © Springer Science+Business Media, LLC 2012

an appropriate cognitive remediation treatment plan. The appendices covering the various tests should help the neuropsychologist gather and interpret the necessary information for developing a plan while the information in the appendices covering NeurXercise helps to determine the exercises most likely to effect cognitive change and generalization of skills.

Appendix A

Attention Domain

Test	Input	Output
Focused Attention		
Digits Forward	Auditory-Numeric	Verbal
Trigrams (0-sec delay)	Auditory-Alphabetic	Verbal
LNNB Rhythm	Auditory-Tonal	Verbal/Motor
Seashore Rhythm	Auditory-Tonal	Verbal
LNNB Word Repetition	Auditory-Verbal	Verbal
Speech Sounds Perception	Auditory-Verbal	Motor
Token Test	Auditory-Verbal	Motor
Spatial Span Forward	Visual-Spatial	Motor
Trails A Sample	Visual-Numeric	Motor
Stroop Color Trial	Visual-Color	Verbal
Stroop Word Trial	Visual-Verbal	Verbal
Sustained Attention		
Conner's CPT	Visual-Verbal	Motor
Running Memory	Visual-Verbal	Motor
VSAT	Visual-Color	Motor
Stroop Color Trial	Visual-Color	Verbal
Stroop Word Trial	Visual-Verbal	Verbal
PASAT	Auditory-Numeric	Verbal
Alternating Attention		
Trails B	Visual-Alphanumeric	Motor
Running Memory	Visual-Verbal	Motor
Conner's CPT	Visual-Verbal	Motor
LNNB	Audiovisual-Verbal	Motor

(continued)

M. H. Podd, *Cognitive Remediation for Brain Injury and Neurological Illness*,
DOI: 10.1007/978-1-4614-1975-4, © Springer Science+Business Media, LLC 2012

(continued)

Test	Input	Output
LNNB Item 6	Auditory-Rhythmic	Motor
Letter Cancellation	Visual-Alphabetic	Motor
Divided Attention		
Trigrams (>0-sec delay)	Auditory-Verbal	Verbal
Digits Backward	Auditory-Numeric	Verbal
Spatial Span Backward	Visual-Spatial	Motor
Selective Attention		
Letter cancellation	Visual-Verbal	Motor
Speech Sounds Perception	Auditory-Tonal	Motor
LNNB Rhythm (old tape)	Auditory-Tonal	Verbal/Motor

Appendix B

Processing Speed

Test	Input	Output
Stroop Color Trial	Visual-Color	Verbal
Stroop Word Trial	Visual-Verbal	Verbal
PASAT	Auditory-Numeric	Verbal
Letter Cancellation	Visual-Verbal	Motor
Trails A	Visual-Numeric	Motor
Conner's CPT	Visual-Verbal	Motor
Running Memory	Visual-Verbal	Motor
LNNB Speed	Visual-Geometric Shapes	Motor
LNNB Speed	Visual-Geometric Shapes	Verbal
LNNB Speed	Auditory-Geometric Shapes	Motor
LNNB Speed	Tactile-Common Objects	Verbal
LNNB Speed	Visual-Pictorial	Verbal
LNNB Speed	Visual-Pictorial	Motor
LNNB Speed	Audiovisual-Verbal	Verbal
LNNB Speed	Auditory	Verbal
LNNB Speed	Visual-Verbal	Verbal
LNNB Speed	Auditory-Numeric	Motor
LNNB Speed	Audioverbal-Numeric	Verbal

M. H. Podd, *Cognitive Remediation for Brain Injury and Neurological Illness*,
DOI: 10.1007/978-1-4614-1975-4, © Springer Science+Business Media, LLC 2012

Appendix C

Perception Domain

Test	Input	Output
Visual scanning and tracking		
Trails A	Visual-Numeric	Motor
Trails B	Visual-Alphanumeric	Motor
VSAT	Visual-Color	Motor
Picture Arrangement	Visual-Pictorial	Motor
Picture Arrangement	Visual-Pictorial	Verbal
Digit Symbol	Visual-Symbolic	Motor
LNNB Picture Sequences	Visual-Pictorial	Verbal/Motor
LNNB Picture Analysis	Visual-Audioverbal	Verbal
Spatial Organization		
LNNB	Visual-Geometric Shapes	Verbal
TPT	Tactile-Geometric Shapes	Motor
Grooved Pegboard	Visual-Spatial	Motor/Spatial
Clock drawings	Verbal	Motor/Spatial
Hooper	Visual	Verbal
Raven's Matrices	Visual	Motor
Porteus Mazes	Visual	Motor
Block Design	Visual	Motor
Object Assembly	Visual	Motor
Rhythm and pitch		
Seashore Rhythm	Auditory-Tonal	Verbal
LNNB Rhythm	Auditory-Tonal	Verbal
LNNB Rhythm	Auditory-Tapping	Motor
LNNB Rhythm	Auditory-Verbal	Motor

M. H. Podd, *Cognitive Remediation for Brain Injury and Neurological Illness*,
DOI: 10.1007/978-1-4614-1975-4, © Springer Science+Business Media, LLC 2012

Appendix D

Sensorimotor Domain

Test	Input	Output
Sensory Perception		
Sensory Perceptual Exam	Tactile	Verbal
Sensory Perceptual Exam	Auditory/Visual	Verbal
TPT	Tactile-Geometric Shapes	Motor
LNNB Tactile	Tactile	Verbal/Motor
Stereognosis		
TPT	Tactile-Geometric Shapes	Motor
Sensory Perceptual Exam	Tactile	Verbal
LNNB Tactile	Tactile	Verbal/Motor
Motor performance		
LNNB Motor	Verbal/Tactile	Motor
Grooved Pegboard	Visual-Spatial	Motor/Spatial
Perdue Pegboard	Visual	Motor
TPT	Tactile-Geometric Shapes	Motor
Finger Tapping	Auditory-Verbal	Motor
Grip Strength	Auditory-Verbal	Motor
Constructional praxis		
Clock drawings	Auditory-Verbal	Motor/Spatial
Aphasia Screening	Auditory-Verbal	Motor
LNNB figure	Visual	Motor
Block Design	Visual	Motor
Visual Reproduction	Visual	Motor
Rey Complex figure	Visual	Motor

M. H. Podd, *Cognitive Remediation for Brain Injury and Neurological Illness*,
DOI: 10.1007/978-1-4614-1975-4, © Springer Science+Business Media, LLC 2012

Appendix E

Language Domain

Test	Input	Output
Expressive speech		
LNNB Expressive Speech	Auditory-Verbal/Visual	Verbal
Aphasia Screening	Auditory-Verbal/Visual	Verbal
Boston Naming	Visual	Verbal
COWAT	Auditory-Verbal	Verbal
Thurstone	Auditory-Verbal	Motor
Receptive Speech		
LNNB Receptive Speech	Auditory-Verbal	Verbal/Motor
Speech Sounds	Auditory-Verbal	Motor
Aphasia Screening	Auditory-Verbal/Visual	Verbal
Token Test	Auditory-Verbal/Visual	Motor

M. H. Podd, *Cognitive Remediation for Brain Injury and Neurological Illness*,
DOI: 10.1007/978-1-4614-1975-4, © Springer Science+Business Media, LLC 2012

Appendix F

Memory Domain

Test	Input	Output
Verbal Memory-Immediate		
Logical Memory I	Auditory-Verbal	Verbal
LNNB Story	Auditory-Verbal	Verbal
CVLT (Trial 1)	Auditory-Verbal	Verbal
AVLT (Trial 1)	Auditory-Verbal	Verbal
LNNB Word List (Trial 1)	Auditory-Verbal	Verbal
WMS III Word List (Trial 1)	Auditory-Verbal	Verbal
Selective Reminding (Trial 1)	Audioverbal/Visual/Spatial	Verbal
Verbal Paired Associates I	Auditory-Verbal	Verbal
Verbal Memory-Under Interference		
AVLT (Trial 6)	Auditory-Verbal	Verbal
CVLT (Trial 6)	Auditory-Verbal	Verbal
LNNB Memory	Auditory-Verbal	Verbal
LNNB Memory	Audioverbal/Audiovisual	Verbal
Trigrams	Auditory-Verbal/Numeric	Verbal
Verbal Memory-Delayed		
Logical Memory II	Auditory-Verbal	Verbal
LNNB Story	Auditory-Verbal	Verbal
CVLT	Auditory-Verbal	Verbal
AVLT	Auditory-Verbal	Verbal
LNNB Word List	Auditory-Verbal	Verbal
WMS III Word List	Auditory-Verbal	Verbal
Cued Selective Reminding	Audioverbal/Visual/Spatial	Verbal
LNNB	Audioverbal/Audiovisual	Verbal/Motor

(continued)

M. H. Podd, *Cognitive Remediation for Brain Injury and Neurological Illness*,
DOI: 10.1007/978-1-4614-1975-4, © Springer Science+Business Media, LLC 2012

(continued)

Test	Input	Output
Verbal Paired Associates II	Auditory-Verbal	Verbal
Nonverbal Memory-Immediate		
TPT	Tactile	Motor
LNNB	Tactile	Verbal
Rey Figure	Visual	Motor
Visual Reproduction I	Visual	Motor
Luria Figure	Visual	Motor
WMS-R Figural Memory	Visual	Motor
Visual Paired Associates I	Visual	Verbal
Nonverbal Memory-Delayed		
TPT	Tactile	Motor
LNNB	Auditory-Verbal	Verbal/Motor
Rey Figure	Visual	Motor
Visual Reproduction II	Visual	Motor
Luria Figure	Visual	Motor
Visual Paired Associates II	Visual	Verbal
Retrieval Method-Free Recall		
Logical Memory II	Auditory-Verbal	Verbal
LNNB Story	Auditory-Verbal	Verbal
CVLT	Auditory-Verbal	Verbal
AVLT	Auditory-Verbal	Verbal
LNNB Word List	Auditory-Verbal	Verbal
WMS III Word List	Auditory-Verbal	Verbal
LNNB	Audioverbal/Audiovisual	Verbal/Motor
TPT	Tactile	Motor
Rey Figure	Visual	Motor
Visual Reproduction II	Visual	Motor
Retrieval Method-Cued Recall		
Selective Reminding	Audioverbal/Visual/Spatial	Verbal
Visual Paired Associates II	Visual	Verbal
Verbal Paired Associates II	Auditory-Verbal	Verbal
Logical Memory II	Visual	Motor
Retrieval Method-Recognition		
AVLT	Visual	Motor
LNNB Delayed Memory	Visual	Verbal
Selective Reminding	Audioverbal/Visual/Spatial	Verbal
Logical Memory II	Visual	Motor
Rey Figure	Visual	Motor
Visual Reproduction II	Visual	Motor
Verbal Paired Associates II	Auditory-Verbal	Verbal
WMS III Word List	Auditory-Verbal	Verbal

Appendix G

Intelligence Domain

Test	Input	Output
Verbal Intelligence		
LNNB Intellectual Processes	Auditory/Visual	Verbal
WAIS III/IV Verbal	Auditory/Visual/Numeric	Verbal
WASI Verbal	Auditory-Verbal	Verbal
SILS Verbal	Auditory-Verbal	Verbal
KBIT	Auditory-Verbal	Verbal
NAART	Visual	Verbal
Barona Index	Auditory or Visual	Verbal or Motor
AFQT	Visual	Motor
Nonverbal Intelligence		
LNNB Intellectual Processes	Auditory-Visual	Verbal/Motor
WAIS III/IV Performance	Visual	Motor
WASI Performance	Visual	Motor
SILS Quantative	Visual	Motor
KBIT	Visual	Motor

M. H. Podd, *Cognitive Remediation for Brain Injury and Neurological Illness*,
DOI: 10.1007/978-1-4614-1975-4, © Springer Science+Business Media, LLC 2012

Appendix H

Academic Domain

LNNB	Audioverbal/Visual-Spatial	Verbal/Motor
WRAT 3/4	Visual	Verbal/Motor
WJ III	Visual/Auditory	Verbal/Motor
WIAT II/III	Visual/Verbal/Auditory	Verbal/Motor

M. H. Podd, *Cognitive Remediation for Brain Injury and Neurological Illness*, DOI: 10.1007/978-1-4614-1975-4, © Springer Science+Business Media, LLC 2012

Appendix I

Executive Functions Domain

Test	Input	Output
Set shifting		
Categories	Visual	Motor
Wisconsin Card Sort	Visual	Motor
Trails B	Visual-Alphanumeric	Motor
Knock/Slap/Chop	Auditory-Verbal	Motor
Teeth/Tongue/Lip	Auditory-Verbal	Oral-Motor
Novelty		
PASAT	Auditory-Numeric	Verbal
Ruff Figural Fluency	Auditory-Verbal	Motor
Problem Solving		
Categories	Visual	Motor
Wisconsin Card Sort	Visual	Motor
SILS Quantitative	Visual	Motor
LNNB Proverbs	Auditory-Verbal	Verbal
LNNB Proverbs	Auditory-Verbal	Verbal/Motor
Block Design	Visual	Motor
Picture Arrangement	Visual	Motor
Problem Solving		
Tower of Hanoi	Visual	Motor
Porteus Mazes	Visual	Motor
LNNB Picture Sequences	Visual	Motor
Impulse Control		
Categories	Visual	Motor
Wisconsin Card Sort	Visual	Motor

(continued)

M. H. Podd, *Cognitive Remediation for Brain Injury and Neurological Illness*,
DOI: 10.1007/978-1-4614-1975-4, © Springer Science+Business Media, LLC 2012

(continued)

Test	Input	Output
Trails B	Visual-Alphanumeric	Motor
PASAT	Auditory-Numeric	Verbal
LNNB Alternating Figure	Visual	Motor
DRS Alternating Figure	Visual	Motor
LNNB Motor Alternation	Visual/Auditory-Verbal	Motor
Trigrams	Auditory-Verbal	Verbal
AVLT	Auditory-Verbal	Verbal
Judgment		
Picture Arrangement	Visual	Motor
Comprehension	Auditory-Verbal	Verbal
LNNB Word List	Auditory-Verbal	Verbal
LNNB Picture Sequences	Visual	Motor

Appendix J

Attention Domain

Exercise	Input	Output
Focused Attention		
Get Q 1	Visual-Alphabetic	Motor
Type It	Visual-Verbal/Alphanumeric	Motor/Verbal
Flasher	Auditory-Tonal	Motor
Flasher	Visual-Color	Motor
Space Probe	Visual-Spatial	Motor
Sustained Attention		
Dartboard	Visual-Spatial	Motor
Run Silent	Visual-Spatial	Motor
Get Q 2 and 3	Visual-Alphabetic	Motor
Two in One	Visual-Verbal	Motor
Alternating Attention		
Get Q 2 and 3	Visual-Alphabetic	Motor
Run Silent 3	Visual-Spatial	Motor
Two in One	Visual-Verbal	Motor
Divided Attention		
Double Trouble 1	Visual-Spatial/Alphabetic	Motor
Double Trouble 2	Visual-Spatial/Audiotonal	Motor

M. H. Podd, *Cognitive Remediation for Brain Injury and Neurological Illness*,
DOI: 10.1007/978-1-4614-1975-4, © Springer Science+Business Media, LLC 2012

Appendix K

Processing Speed

Exercise	Input	Output
Get Q	Visual-Alphabetic	Motor
Two in One	Visual-Verbal	Motor
Dartboard	Visual-Spatial	Motor
Invaders	Visual-Spatial	Motor
Run Silent 1 and 2	Visual-Spatial	Motor

M. H. Podd, *Cognitive Remediation for Brain Injury and Neurological Illness*,
DOI: 10.1007/978-1-4614-1975-4, © Springer Science+Business Media, LLC 2012

Appendix L

Perception Domain

Exercise	Input	Output
Visual scanning and tracking		
Get Q	Visual-Alphabetic	Motor
Space Probe	Visual-Spatial	Motor/Spatial
Dartboard	Visual-Spatial	Motor/Spatial
Run Silent	Visual-Spatial	Motor/Spatial
Invaders	Visual-Spatial	Motor/Spatial
Bomber	Visual-Spatial	Motor/Spatial
Spatial Organization		
Flasher	Visual-Color	Motor
Flasher	Auditory-Tonal	Motor
Run Silent	Visual-Spatial	Motor/Spatial
Invaders	Visual-Spatial	Motor/Spatial
Strategy	Visual-Verbal	Motor-Spatial
Hid in the Grid	Visual-Spatial	Motor/Spatial
Concentration 1	Visual-Pictorial	Motor/Spatial
Concentration 2	Visual-Facial	Motor/Spatial
Towers of Hanoi	Visual-Spatial	Motor/Spatial
Map Reading	Visual-Spatial/Visual-Verbal	Motor
Detective 1	Visual-Facial	Motor
Detective 2	Visual-Verbal	Motor
Golf	Visual-Verbal	Motor
Two in One 3 and 4	Visual-Verbal	Motor

M. H. Podd, *Cognitive Remediation for Brain Injury and Neurological Illness*,
DOI: 10.1007/978-1-4614-1975-4, © Springer Science+Business Media, LLC 2012

Appendix M

Memory Domain

Exercise	Input	Output
Verbal Memory-Immediate		
Memory Game 1	Visual-Alphabetic	Motor
Memory Game 2	Visual-Verbal	Motor
Foreign Intrigue 2	Visual-Alphabetic	Motor
Foreign Intrigue 3	Visual-Verbal	Motor
Shopping List	Visual-Verbal	Motor
Verbal Memory-Under Interference		
Memory Game 2	Visual-Verbal	Motor
Verbal Memory-Delayed		
Buying Power 3	Visual-Verbal/Numeric	Motor
Nonverbal Memory-Immediate		
Flasher	Visual-Color	Motor
Flasher	Auditory-Tonal	Motor
Concentration 1	Visual-Pictorial	Motor/Spatial
Concentration 2	Visual-Facial	Motor/Spatial
Symbol Memory	Visual-Symbolic	Motor
Line Up	Visual-Facial	Motor
Foreign Intrigue 1	Visual-Facial	Motor
Nonverbal Memory-Delayed		
Concentration 1	Visual-Pictorial	Motor/Spatial
Concentration 2	Visual-Facial	Motor/Spatial
Line Up	Visual-Facial	Motor
Time Travel	Visual-Facial	Motor

(continued)

(continued)

Exercise	Input	Output
Retrieval Method-Free Recall		
Memory Game 1	Visual-Alphabetic	Motor
Memory Game 2	Visual-Verbal	Motor
Shopping List	Visual-Verbal	Motor
Flasher	Visual-Color	Motor
Flasher	Auditory-Tonal	Motor
Concentration 1	Visual-Pictorial	Motor/Spatial
Concentration 2	Visual-Facial	Motor/Spatial
Time Travel 2	Visual-Facial	Motor
Retrieval Method-Cued Recall		
What's My Name	Visual/Visual-Verbal	Verbal/Motor
Symbol Memory	Visual-Symbolic	Motor
Retrieval Method-Recognition		
Foreign Intrigue 1	Visual-Facial	Motor
Foreign Intrigue 2	Visual-Alphabetic	Motor
Foreign Intrigue 3	Visual-Verbal	Motor
Time Travel 1	Visual-Facial	Motor
Line Up	Visual-Facial	Motor

Appendix N

Executive Functions Domain

Exercise	Input	Output
Set shifting		
Mission Decode	Visual	Motor
Detective 1	Visual-Facial	Motor
Detective 2	Visual-Verbal	Motor
Two in One	Visual-Verbal	Motor
Get Q 2 and 3	Visual-Alphabetic	Motor
Run Silent 3	Visual-Spatial	Motor/Spatial
Double Trouble 1	Visual/Visual-Alphabetic	Motor/Spatial
Double Trouble 2	Visual/Auditory-Tonal	Motor/Spatial
Problem Solving: Reasoning and Convergent/Divergent Thinking		
Mission Decode	Visual	Motor
Detective 1	Visual-Facial	Motor
Detective 2	Visual-Verbal	Motor
Vocabulary	Visual-Verbal	Motor
Strategy 2 and 3	Visual-Spatial	Motor/Spatial
Spies	Visual-Facial	Motor
Problem Solving: Planning Ahead		
Strategy 3	Visual-Spatial	Motor/Spatial
Invaders	Visual-Spatial	Motor/Spatial
Map Reading	Visual-Verbal	Motor
Towers of Hanoi	Visual-Spatial	Motor
Run Silent 3	Visual-Spatial	Motor/Spatial
Number Guesser	Visual-Numeric	Motor
Hid in the Grid	Visual-Spatial	Motor/Spatial

(continued)

M. H. Podd, *Cognitive Remediation for Brain Injury and Neurological Illness*,
DOI: 10.1007/978-1-4614-1975-4, © Springer Science+Business Media, LLC 2012

(continued)

Exercise	Input	Output
Impulse Control		
Mission Decode	Visual	Motor
Detective 1	Visual-Facial	Motor
Detective 2	Visual-Verbal	Motor
Vocabulary	Visual-Verbal	Motor
Two in One	Visual-Verbal	Motor
Get Q	Visual-Alphabetic	Motor
Run Silent	Visual-Spatial	Motor/Spatial
Invaders	Visual-Spatial	Motor/Spatial
Body Language 2	Visual	Motor
Judgment		
Body Language	Visual	Motor
Vocabulary	Visual-Verbal	Motor
Mission Decode	Visual	Motor
Detective 1	Visual-Facial	Motor
Detective 2	Visual-Verbal	Motor
Spies	Visual-Facial	Motor

References

Alexander, M. P. (1995). Mild traumatic brain injury: Pathophysiology, natural history, and clinical management. *Neurology, 45,* 1253–1260.

Almi, C. R., & Finger, S. (1992). Brain injury and recovery of function: Theories and Mechanisms of functional reorganization.*Journal of Head Trauma Rehabilitation, 7*(2), 70–77.

American Psychiatric Association. (2000). *Diagnostic and statistical manual of mental disorders* (4th ed.). Text revision. Washington DC: Author.

Barkley, R. A., Fischer, M., Smallish, L., & Fletcher, K. (2002). The persistence of attention-deficit/hyperactivity disorder into young adulthood as a function of reporting source and definition of disorder. *Journal of Abnormal Psychology, 111,* 279–289.

Benton, A., & Tranel, D. (1993). Visuoperceptual, visuospatial, and visuoconstructive disorders. In K. M. Heilman & E. Vallenstein (Eds.), *Clinical Neuropsychology* (3rd ed., pp. 165–213). New York: Oxford.

Ben-Yishay, Y., Piasetsky, E. B., & Rattok, J. (1987). A systematic method for ameliorating disorders in basic attention. In M. J. Meier, A. L. Benton & L. Diller, (Eds.), *Neuropsychological Rehabilitation* (pp. 165–181). New York: Guilford Press.

Belanger, H. G., Curtiss, G., Demery, J. A., Lebowitz, B. K., & Vanderploeg, R. D. (2005). Factors moderating neuropsychological outcomes following mild traumatic brain injury: A meta-analysis. *Journal of the International Neuropsychological Society, 11*(3), 215–227.

Bigler, E. D. (2008). Neuropsychology and clinical neuroscience of persistent post concussive syndrome.*Journal of the International Neuropsychological Society, 14,* 1–22.

Binder, L. M., Rohling, M. L., Larrabee, G. J. (1997). A review of mild head trauma. Meta-analytic review of neuropsychological studies. *Journal of Clinical and Experimental Neuropsychology, 19,* 421–431

Bracy, O. L. (1985). *Programs for Cognitive Rehabilitation.* Indianapolis, IN: Psychological Software Services.

Broca, P. (1865). Du Siege de la faculte du language articule. *Bulletin of the Society of Anthropology, 6,* 377–393.

Caruso, L.S., & Ash, A. (2007). Multiple sclerosis and cognition: Implications for cognitive rehabilitation. Division of Neuropsychology *Newsletter 40, 25*(2), 3-11.

Christensen, J., Pedeersen, M. G., Pedersen, C. B., Sidenius, P., Olsen, J., & Vestergaard, M. (2009). Long-term risk of epilepsy after traumatic brain injury in children and young Adults: A population-based cohort study. *Lancet, 373,* 1105–1110.

Christodoulou, C. (2005). Neuroimaging of cognitive dysfunction in multiple sclerosis with multiple magnetic resonance measures. Division of Clinical Neuropsychology *Newsletter 40, 23*(1), 11–14.

M. H. Podd, *Cognitive Remediation for Brain Injury and Neurological Illness,*   153
DOI: 10.1007/978-1-4614-1975-4, © Springer Science+Business Media, LLC 2012

Cicerone, K. D., Dahlberg, C., Kalmar, K., Langenbahn, D. M., Malec, J. F., Bergquist, T. F., et al. (2000). Evidence-based cognitive rehabilitation: Recommendations for clinical practice. *Archives of Physical Medicine Rehabilitation, 81*, 1596–1615.

Cicerone,K. D., Dahlberg, C., Malec, J. F., Langenbaum, D. M., Felicett, T., Kniepp, S., Ellmo, W., Kalmar, K., Giacino, J. T., Harley, J. P., Laatsch, L., Morse, P. A., & Catanese, J. (2005) Evidence-based cognitive rehabilitation: Updated review of the literature from 1998 to 2002.

Cicerone, K. D. (2002). Remediation of 'working attention' in mild traumatic brain injury. *Brain injury, 16*, 185–195.

Craine, G. F., & Gudeman, H. E. (1981). *The rehabilitation of brain functions: Principles procedures and techniques of neurotraining.* Springfield, IL: Charles C. Thomas.

Denney, D. R., Sworowski, L. A., & Lynch, S. G. (2005). Cognitive impairment in three subtypes of multiple sclerosis. *Archives of Clinical Neuropsychology, 20*, 967–981.

Filley, C. M., Heaton, R. K., Thompson, L. L., Nelson, L. M., & Franklin, G. M. (1990). Effects of disease course on neuropsychological functioning. In S. M. Rao (Ed.), *Neurobehavioral aspects of multiple sclerosis* (pp. 139–148). New York: Oxford.

Frencham, K. A., Fox, A. M., & Mayberry, M. T. (2005). Neuropsychological studies of mild traumatic brain injury: a meta-analytic review of research since 1995. *Journal of Clinical and Experimental Neuropsychology, 27*(3), 334–351.

French, L. M., Spector, J., Stiers, W., & Kane, R. L. (2010). Blast injury and traumatic Brain Injury. In C. H. Kennedy and J. L. Moore (Eds.), *Military neuropsychology* (pp. 101–125). New York: Springer Publishing Company.

Garlaza, K. O., Fulmer, J., Burns, W. J., & Montgomery, D. (1999). *Cognitive training and seriously disturbed children,* August. Poster presented at the annual meeting of the American Psychological Association, Boston, MA.

Germano, G. D., Capellini, S. A. (2008) Efficacy of an audio-visual computerized remediation program in students with dyslexia. *Pró-Fono Revista de Atualização Científica 20*(4), 237–242

Gianutsos, R., & Klitzner, C. (1981). *Computer Programs for Cognitive Remediation.* Bayport, NY: Life Sciences Associates.

Golden, C.J., Purisch, A.D. & Hammeke, T.A (1979/1995). *Luria-Nebraska Neuropsychological Battery: Manual* Los Angeles: Western Psychological Services.

Golden, C. J., Moses, J. A., Coffman, J. A., Miller, W. R., & Strider, F. D. (1983). *Clinical Neuropsychology: Interface with neurologic and psychiatric disorders.* New York: Grune & Stratton.

Golden, C. J., Warren, W. L., & Espe-Pfeiffer, P. (1999). *LNNB Handbook: 20th Anniversary.* Los Angeles: Western Psychological Services.

Goldstein, K. (1939). *The Organism.* New York: American Book.

Greiffenstein, M. F. (2003). The case for the case study. National Academy of Neuropsychology Bulletin, *18*(2), 5, 17.

Hall, E. D., Sullivan, P. G., Gibson, T. R., Pavel, K. M., Thompson, B. M., & Scheff, S. W. (2005). Spatial and temporal characteristics of neurodegeneration after controlled cortical impact in mice: More than a focul brain injury. *Journal of Neurotrauma, 22*, 252–265.

Heilman, K. M. (2002). *Matter of mind: A neurologist's view of brain-behavior Relationships.* New York: Oxford.

Hervey, A. S., Epstein, J. N., & Curry, J. F. (2004). Neuropsychology of adults with attention-deficit/hyperactivity disorder: A meta-analytic review. *Neuropsychology, 18*(3), 485–503.

Julian, L. J. (2007). Cognitive dusfunction in the earliest stages of multiple sclerosis. *Division of Neuropsychology Newsletter 40, 25 (2), 1*(12), 17–22.

Kashluba, S., Paniak, C., & Casey, J. E. (2008). Persisitent symptoms associated with factors identified by the WHO task force on mild traumatic brain injury. *Clinical Neuropsychology, 22*, 195–208.

Klonoff, P. S., Olson, K. C., Talley, M. C., Husk, K. L., Myles, S. M., Gehrels, J. A., et al. (2010). The relationship of cognitive retraining to neurological patients' driving status: The role of process variables and compensation training. *Brain Injury, 24*(2), 63–73.

References

Klonoff, P. S., Talley, M.c., Dawson, L. K., Myles, S. M., Watt, L. M., Gehrels, J. A., et al. (2007). The relationship of cognitive retraining to neurological patients' work and school status. *Brain Injury, 21*(11), 1097–1107.

Lashley, K. S. (1938). Factors limiting recovery after central nervous system lesions. *Journal of Nervous and Mental Diseases, 88,* 733–755.

Lezak, M. D. (1995). *Neuropsychological Assessment:* (3rd ed.). New York: Oxford.

Luria, A. R. (1962;1966). *Higher cortical functions in man.* New York: Basic Books.

Luria, A. R. (1948;1963). *Restoration of function after brain injury.* New York: Pergamon.

Luria, A. R. (1973). *The working brain.* New York: Basic Books.

Luria, A. R. (1980). *Higher cortical functions in man* (2nd ed.). New York: Basic Books.

Lynch, W. J. (1979). *A Guide to Atari Home Computer Programs for Rehabilitation Settings.* Palo Alto: Author.

MacDonald, C. L., Johnson, A. M., Cooper, D., Nelson, E. C., Werner, N. J., Shimony, J. S., et al. (2011). Detection of blast-related traumatic brain injury in U.S. military personnel. The New England Journal of Medicine, *364*(22), 2091–2100.

McCrae, M. A. (2007). *Mild traumatic brain injury and postconcussion syndrome: The new evidence base for diagnosis and treatment.* New York: Oxford.

Moses, J. A., & Maruish, M. E. (1990). A critical review of the Luria-Nebraska Neuropsychological Battery literature: XI. *Critiques and rebuttals. Part Two. International Journal of Clinical Neuropsychology, 12*(1), 37–45.

Moses, J. A., & Maruish, M. E. (1991). A critical review of the Luria-Nebraska Neuropsychological Battery literature: XIV. *Retrospect and Prospect.International Journal of Clinical Neuropsychology, 13*(3–4), 178–188.

NIH. (1999). *Report of the NIH consensus development conference on the rehabilitation of persons with traumatic brain injury.* Bethesda: National Institutes of Health.

Povlishock, J.T. & Katz, D.I. (2005). Update of neuropathology and neurological recovery after traumatic brain injury. *Jouranl of Head Trauma Rehabilitation, 20,* 76–94

Pertab, J. L., James, K. M., & Bigler, E. D. (2009). Limitations of mild traumatic brain injury meta-analyses. *Brain Injury, 23*(6), 498–508.

Podd, M. H., Krehbiel, M. A., Reeves, D. L., Miller, J., & House, J. (1996, November). *Maintenance of beneficial effects of cognitive remediation: post treatment follow up of attentional gains. Poster presented at the meeting of the National Academy of Neuropsychology,* New Orleans, LA.

Podd, M. H. (1998a). *Successful cognitive remediation of moderate/severe brain injury: Three case studies.* Poster presented at National Academy of Neuropsychology, Washington, DC.

Podd, M. H. (1998b). *Successful treatment of patients with extraordinary premorbid visual memory: Three Case studies.* Poster presented at National Academy of Neuropsychology, Washington, DC.

Podd, M. H. (1998c). *Changes in performance on the Luria-Nebraska Neuropsychological Battery following cognitive remediation.* Presentation at National Academy of Neuropsychology, Washington, DC.

Podd, M. H. (2000). *The cognitive remediation for MS and right frontal meningioma resection.* Williamsberg, VA: Paper presented at.

Podd and Krehbiel (2006). *Return to work rate and improved neuropsychological test performance as a function of inclusion of cognitive remediation for attentional deficits in the treatment plan.* Unpublished manuscript.

Podd, M. H., & Seelig, D. P. (1989). *NeurXerxise manual.* Fort Washington: neurX.

Podd, M. H., & Seelig, D. P. (1994). *NeurXerxise manual.* Fort Washington: neurX.

Podd, M. H., & Seelig, D. P. (1999). *Building a neuropsychology practice: A guide to respecialization.* Northvale: Jason Aronson.

Ponsford, J.L., & Kinsella, G. (1988). Evaluation of a remedial programme for attentional deficits following closed head injury. *Journal of Clinical and Experimental Neuropsychology, 10,* 693–708.

Stein, D.G., Brailowsky, S. & Will, B. (1995). *Brain repair*. New York: Oxford.

Stuss, D.T.,Stethem, L.L. & Poirier, C.A. (1987), Comparison of three tests of attention and rapid information processing across six age groups. *The Clinical Neuropsychologist, 1*, 139–152.

Vanderploeg, R. D., Belanger, H. G., & Curtiss, G. (2009). Mild traumatic brain injury and posttraumatic stress disorder and their associations with health symptoms. *Archives of Physical Medicine and Rehabilitation, 90*(7), 1084–1093.

Vanderploeg, R. D., Curtiss, G., & Belanger, H. G. (2005). Long-term neuropsychological outcomes following mild traumatic brain injury. *Journal of the International Neuropsychological Society, 11*(3), 228–236.

Von Monakow, C. (1914/1960). Localization of brain functions. In *Some papers on the cerebral cortex*, Springfield, IL: Charles C. Thomas

Von Wild, K. R. H. (2008). Posttraumatic rehabilitation and one year outcome following acute traumatic brain injury (TBI): Data from the well defined population based German prospective study 2000–2002. *Acta Neurochirgica Supplementum, 101*, 55–60.

Wernicke, K. (1874). Der aphasische Symptomenkomplex. Breslau Translated in *Boston Studies in Philosophy of Science, 4*, 34–97.

Wiederholt, W. C. (1982). *Neurology for non-neurologists*. New York: Academic Press.

Index

M. H. Podd, *Cognitive Remediation for Brain Injury and Neurological Illness*,   157
DOI: 10.1007/978-1-4614-1975-4, © Springer Science+Business Media, LLC 2012